POSTCARD HISTORY SERIES

Sanatoriums and Asylums of Eastern North Carolina

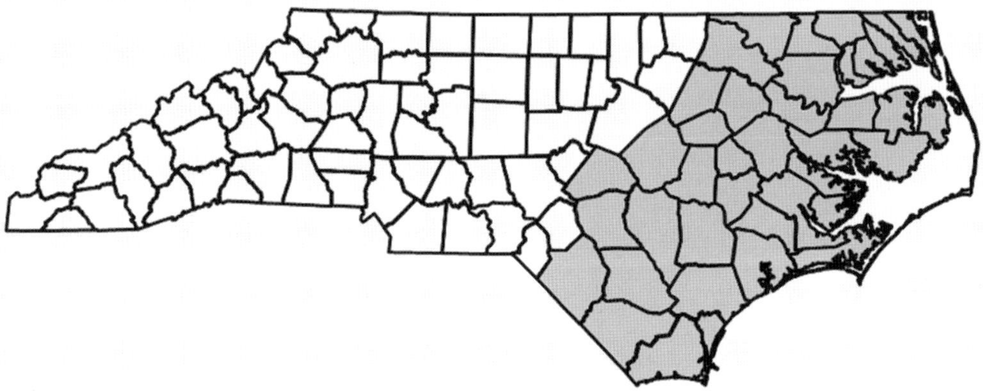

North Carolina is comprised of 100 counties. North to south, the state is rather narrow, but east to west, the differences are distinct, ranging from geography to climate. For this work, Eastern North Carolina includes those counties along the Interstate 95 corridor and all points east. (Photography by author.)

On the Front Cover: The S.R. Fowle Memorial Hospital opened in 1902 in Washington. The hospital stood at the site now occupied by the Washington Fire Department. It was founded by a group of doctors, including Dr. Edwin Brown. In 1923, the 30-bed hospital was led by Dr. John L. Nicholson. (Author's personal collection.)

On the Back Cover: The James Walker Memorial Hospital opened in 1901 at the site of the old City/County Hospital. James Walker was a stonemason, contractor, and builder. He came to Wilmington after being awarded the contract to build the US Marine Hospital there in 1856. One of his later projects included the Western North Carolina Sanatorium. He died three months before his final project, the James Walker Memorial Hospital, opened. (Author's personal collection.)

POSTCARD HISTORY SERIES

Sanatoriums and Asylums of Eastern North Carolina

Dr. Randy D. Kearns

ARCADIA PUBLISHING

ISBN 978-1-4671-2858-2

Published by Arcadia Publishing
Charleston, South Carolina

Printed in the United States of America

Library of Congress Control Number: 2017955984

For all general information contact Arcadia Publishing at:
Telephone 843-853-2070
Fax 843-853-0044
E-mail sales@arcadiapublishing.com
For customer service and orders:
Toll-Free 1-888-313-2665

Visit us on the Internet at www.arcadiapublishing.com

This book is dedicated to my wife, Kristin;
our children Josh, Katie, and Kendahl;
and my late parents, Edgar and Ida Kearns.

Contents

Acknowledgments

Postcards at the dawn of the 20th century were akin to the email or text message of today. They were a frequent form of quick and relatively inexpensive communication. These cards offer a glimpse into the past with images long since forgotten or forever altered by nature or man.

Many of the postcards included are 80–115 years old. Several more are relatively newer, but all reveal the transition of regional health care. Most of the photographers and postcard publishers are of a bygone era, but it is through their tireless efforts, these images are available today.

Images are either part of the author's personal collection or commonly found archived on digital sites operated by East Carolina University; the North Carolina Digital Library; UNC Libraries; New Hanover County Library; Wilson County Public Library; Craven County Public Library; or the North Carolina Collection Photographic Archives, Wilson Library, UNC-Chapel Hill. A special thanks to those who helped track down materials for this work, including the North Carolina State Archives, New Hanover County Public Library, Wilson County Public Library, Sheppard Memorial Library Greenville, Wayne County Public Library, Martin County Public Library, the *State Port Pilot* newspaper, Arthur Brown Jr. for sharing his family archives of hospital materials, and Kenneth Lee Coleman Jr. for the Roseboro Hospital information.

Several of the specific details regarding these great buildings were sourced from a large hospital registry database first compiled by the American Medical Association (AMA) in 1906. The AMA relied on a postcard to conduct the polling with an example included (page 126). A massive (approximately 2,500 pages) book was created and versions referenced throughout this work include significant details such as locations, specific dates, capacity, and capabilities. This included the facility physician in charge (PIC).

It should also be noted that there are a variety of spellings for several towns to include: Goldsboro/Goldsborough, New Bern/Newbern/Newberne, Averasboro/Averasborough, and Tarboro/Tarborough. Several towns have changed names: Smithville to Southport, Toisnot to Elm City, and Duke to Erwin.

Several words used in this text solely reflect their historical context. These terms include demeaning words such as "retarded" and "negro." Those terms are examples of a past we should neither celebrate nor forget.

This book was created by an academic with a target audience of those who are interested in the images of our past, with the hope that everyone will support the preservation of that history. Please consider your support of the historical societies and other organizations dedicated to the preservation of our past.

Introduction

Eastern North Carolina has a unique history that includes witnessing the arrival of the first English explorers to the New World and the home of the first governor of the Carolina Colony. The region includes multiple shipping ports, railroads, and cities in a state with a great climate. As the regional population grew, so did the need for medical care. The earliest documentation of medical care being provided and compensated by the church occurred in Edenton in 1703 by Dr. Godfrey Spruill.

Before the cause and management of infectious disease was clearly understood and a cure discovered, the best care included rest, fresh air, and good nutrition, all under the watchful eye of a trained medical professional. The asylums and sanitoriums were places of refuge and recovery. Long before we understood the science, we understood the need for rest, personal attention, and good nutrition.

The emergence of the insane asylums and feeblemindedness institutions began in the 19th century. For those considered insane, proper medical care meant institutionalization at an asylum. "Lunatic asylum" was used to describe the first permanent buildings constructed for those considered mentally ill (or insane) to be managed and kept safe. ("Madhouse" was more commonly used in Europe at the time.) By the early 20th century, an effort was under way to separately manage those who were mentally ill from those considered "retarded" or "feebleminded" (the term "special needs" is more commonly used today). Nevertheless, the differences remained poorly understood well into the 20th century.

The large institutions (asylums and sanatoriums) were typically created and operated by a government (in this case, the State of North Carolina). While governmental funding was received annually, these institutions made significant strides toward being self-sufficient. The healthier or more able-bodied patients, along with the staff, maintained a farm that produced meat, fruit, and vegetables. Several institutions sold their excess milk and vegetables to support the cost of the facility further. All needed to raise money through a variety of methods to support the operation.

Sanitas is Latin for "health," and *sanus* means "healthy, sane." The English derivative offers the word "sanatorium." A sanatorium was a broader term used to describe these buildings where patients were taken for the treatment of various chronic diseases but more often was specific to managing tuberculosis. Eastern North Carolina was an ideal location for a sanatorium with its mild climate and proximity to a variety of ocean ports and railroads, which provided reliable transportation. Other contributing factors for locating a sanatorium included access to fresh air, the scent of a vast pine forest, or healing springs. The treatment and healing process was long and extensive, but these facilities typically positioned the patient to allow the body to recover from the infection.

The spelling variations of the word "sanatorium" can be seen on the actual card and facility signage in the images throughout this book. Other spellings include sanitorium, sanatarium, sanitarium, and sanatoria. Although the variation "sanitarium" was more commonly used to describe a "health resort," the words were commonly interchanged. Occasionally, these facilities were also referred to as institutions.

Plagues and pandemics ravaged much of Europe between the 14th and 18th centuries, which spurred the growth of medicine. The method that emerged as the best way to manage the sick patients and stop the spread of disease was to separate the sick patients (those with an infectious disease) away from the public in a building known as a pesthouse. However, a French word, *lazaretto*, was also used when the lines blurred between a pesthouse and quarantine stations. The origin of the pesthouse is associated with the bubonic plague. Typical outbreaks in Eastern North Carolina included yellow fever and smallpox. Pesthouse was the more commonly used word during the 19th century. However, by the early 20th century, this place became increasingly known as the sanatorium for those with infections needing long-term care.

The almshouse is a charity-supported, long-term care home. The almshouse usually included a hospital or infirmary for those residents with chronic health issues. The almshouse typically served a specific group of people such as veterans, orphans, widows of veterans, the destitute, or a common former employer such as railroad retirees. If supported by the local government, a colloquial name for the almshouse was the "county home" or the "poor folk's home." Fraternal organizations also operated almshouses. These organizations included the Independent Order of the Odd Fellows and Rebekahs, the Elks, the Free Masons, and various church or religious groups.

The word *hospital* is a Latin derivative of "hospitalia," meaning a place where strangers were received and provided care. In Greek mythology, the son of the god Apollo was Asclepius. The symbol typically used in medicine—a staff with the serpent wrapped around it (the healing stick)—is associated with him. Built for Asclepius in 430 BC, the temple at Epidaurus, where the sick or injured would spend the night, became the healing shrine. The Greek physician Hippocrates (all physicians today take the Hippocratic Oath) was an Asclepiad. In time, the temple at Epidaurus grew to 180 rooms, taking in the sick and injured as well as women in childbirth.

Hospital first appears in Roman literature describing a place in a military camp where injured soldiers were treated. Hospitals were also erected for sick slaves and gladiators. During fourth-century Rome, civilian hospitals were erected as a function of Christian churches after the Council of Nicaea in 325 AD. Fourteen centuries later, the word hospital remained a temporary place where soldiers were cared for as wars raged, or a more permanent location for travelers, mariners, and the destitute. During the 18th, and 19th centuries, most illness and injury continued to be managed in the home with doctors making their home visits.

This remained the case during the American Revolutionary War and most notably the American Civil War. Both included multiple hospitals in fixed locations as well as those that were mobile as great armies moved across Eastern North Carolina.

War wounds and infectious diseases almost equally contributed to the mortality and morbidity of soldiers. The spread of disease was poorly understood and the value of hygiene seldom appreciated. While there were noted efforts to separate the sick (in pesthouses) from the injured (in hospitals), this was infrequent. Approximately 40,000 North Carolinian Confederate soldiers died, with almost half of the death rate attributed to disease. The most common diseases included diarrhea, dysentery (also called blood flux), typhoid fever, erysipelas (an acute infectious disease of the skin and mucous membranes accompanied by fever and caused by streptococcus), pneumonia, measles, smallpox, malaria, tuberculosis, and scurvy. This list reflects the inadequate food supply as well as the poor sanitation and hygiene practices throughout the encampments.

War injuries typically involved a gunshot wound. These wounds were produced by firing a minié ball (bullet) from a pistol or rifle at a low velocity (for a firearm). As the bullet pierced the skin, it would take with it a small piece of clothing. Uniforms were worn for long periods of time without regular cleaning. Surgeons would probe the wound. Recovering the bullet and the cloth was essential to reduce infection-related mortality. If the arm or leg was shot, an expeditious solution was to amputate. Surgeons became skilled in quickly amputating the injured limb just above the wound. In the years after the war, significant portions of state budgets were used to purchase artificial limbs for the veterans.

Aside from war, the first US hospitals were built for sailors/seamen and mariners as they arrived in port either sick or injured and nowhere near home. The US Marine Hospitals were constructed at or near major shipping ports. For the general population, the country doctor was summoned to visit the ill or injured and typically cared for in their homes by family members.

Over the past 100 years, Eastern North Carolina became the home of major military bases with air and sea access. During the world wars, large hospitals were constructed nearby to manage the thousands of injured soldiers evacuated from Europe. After the wars, the ongoing health care needs of the returning veterans were served at hospitals and clinics built by the US Veterans Administration.

General hospitals began to emerge in the early 20th century. They were constructed for those patients with little or no family support to care for them if they were sick or injured. These hospitals were often affiliated with a church or community group. As the 20th century began, racial segregation, particularly in Southern states, led to the "separate but equal" approach for many services, including health care. While some hospitals had "colored wards," others were whites only. "Colored or negro" hospitals emerged to meet the need.

By early to mid-20th century, clinics in small communities took on larger roles by adding beds for patients who needed to be treated overnight, typically when a hospital was not in the area. These clinics were commonly referred to as either a hospital, a clinic, or both. If these clinics or hospitals were part of a larger complex operation such as a university or orphanage, they were called infirmaries. The infirmary typically met the definition of a hospital. When Medicare and Medicaid emerged as the principal payment source, rules associated with receiving payment for care forced these small facilities to either shed their overnight services or grow into a hospital.

The temporary hospital emerged as a place of care during wars and disasters. The quarantine camp or lazaretto was created during pandemics or local/regional disease outbreaks. The temporary hospitals were created in adapted spaces or hastily constructed buildings near transportation resources such as trains, ocean ports, and airports. With large infectious disease outbreaks such as influenza, smallpox, yellow fever, and polio, a variety of buildings supplemented by tents have been used. With the looming threat of nuclear war, the US civil defense effort included hundreds of temporary hospital packages distributed across the country. Another variation of the temporary hospital emerged after the September 11, 2001, terrorist attacks.

Several of the more significant changes for the health care profession were influenced by science, funding changes, or new laws regulating the profession. While the Lunacy Act (1845) became law in England, its influence was global. The act coincided with the tireless efforts of a mental health champion, Dorothea Lynde Dix, who arrived in North Carolina in 1848. Dix convinced North Carolina leaders to construct an institution (which opened in 1856, named in her honor).

The first records of providing care and comfort to a sick patient can be traced to Edenton in 1703, including "Doc" Godfrey Spruill leading an effort to nurse a patient back to health. The role of the nurse was more abstract but came into focus particularly in the American Civil War. The link of hygiene and infection was poorly understood at the time. However, a nurse by the name of Florence Nightingale applied her war experiences (from the Crimea Wars) to a book she penned in 1859 called *Notes in Nursing*. While her home was London, her work was critically influential as American Civil War hospitals were overwhelmed with injured and ill soldiers.

The role of the nurse became more specific in the American Civil War, and nurses became essential in the hospital during the years that followed. By the turn of the 20th century, nurse training programs were emerging alongside hospitals and sanatoriums at places like Wilson

Sanatorium, Mercy Hospital, Highsmith Hospital, and the James Walker Memorial Hospital. Led by the efforts of Mary Lewis Wyche, the North Carolina Legislature enacted the nation's first Nurse Practice Act (1903).

The Flexner Report (1910) was sanctioned by the Carnegie Foundation to explore the quality of an American medical education. The Flexner Report was credited with improving the quality of medical education. Critics, however, question just how much should be attributed to the report and point out the widespread closure of "colored only" medical schools following the report. (All but two of the "colored only" medical schools closed in the years following the report.)

The Hospital Survey and Construction Act (also known as the Hill-Burton Act) was signed into law by Pres. Harry Truman in 1946. Hill-Burton funding led to the construction of new hospitals and modernization of existing hospitals across Eastern North Carolina. The funding included grants and loans with a requirement that the facility provides care for patients regardless of ability to pay. These hospitals were typically owned by the local government, the church, or the community. Rural communities, which sorely lacked adequate health care, benefited greatly from Hill-Burton funding.

Scientific discovery led to the closure of the sanatorium. Consumption, Pott's Disease, and the white plague were terms used at one point or another to describe the deadly disease known as tuberculosis (TB). In 1943, two graduate students at Rutgers University discovered streptomycin. While a TB vaccine was first used on a human in 1921, it was not until the early 1950s that the vaccine and a cure (streptomycin) were widely being used to diminish the disease rapidly. By 1960, the sanitorium had either closed or evolved into a hospital.

The passage of the Civil Rights Act in 1964 and amendments to the Social Security Act in 1965 created and shaped Medicare and Medicaid. These changes resulted in two substantial health care evolutions. Medicare and Medicaid provided the first reliable cash flow for hospitals for services rendered. The new programs also included antidiscrimination requirements for participating in the Medicare and Medicaid payment programs, thus leading to the demise of segregated health care. During the 1960s–1980s, many smaller hospitals either consolidated or closed, giving way to the construction of more comprehensive and modern hospitals.

The passage of the Balanced Budget Act of 1997 included substantial cuts to funding for health care in general and hospitals specifically. The concern for the safety of particularly small hospitals in rural communities led to the insertion of a provision to create a Critical Access Hospital (CAH) designation. The CAH designation protected funding for small hospitals (less than 25 staffed beds) that solely serve rural communities and are not otherwise served by larger medical centers. Given the rural nature for much of Eastern North Carolina, this has been a lifesaver for several hospitals but not enough for others.

One

Mental Illness (Insane Asylum) Versus Mental Retardation

The lunatic asylum (also known as the madhouse) became the hospital for those who struggled to live in a society without great accommodation or peril. The board of directors for the North Carolina Insane Asylum, led by Dr. Edmund Burke Haywood, urged the North Carolina General Assembly (NCGA) to develop asylums for Western North Carolina as well as one for the "blacks of the state." The NCGA appointed a committee to identify and recommend a site for the construction of a state asylum that would serve the mentally ill patients of color. A location of just under 200 acres near Goldsboro was purchased in April 1878, and construction began shortly thereafter.

Dr. Ira Hardy's family, of LaGrange, included a child with special needs. He described the condition as "feeblemindedness" or "mentally retarded." His paper, "What It Costs," presented to the Seaboard Medical Society, led to a movement to create the Feeble-Minded Institute, which opened in Kinston in 1912. Today, the facility is known as the Caswell Center (renamed to honor a Kinston area native and North Carolina's first governor, Richard Caswell).

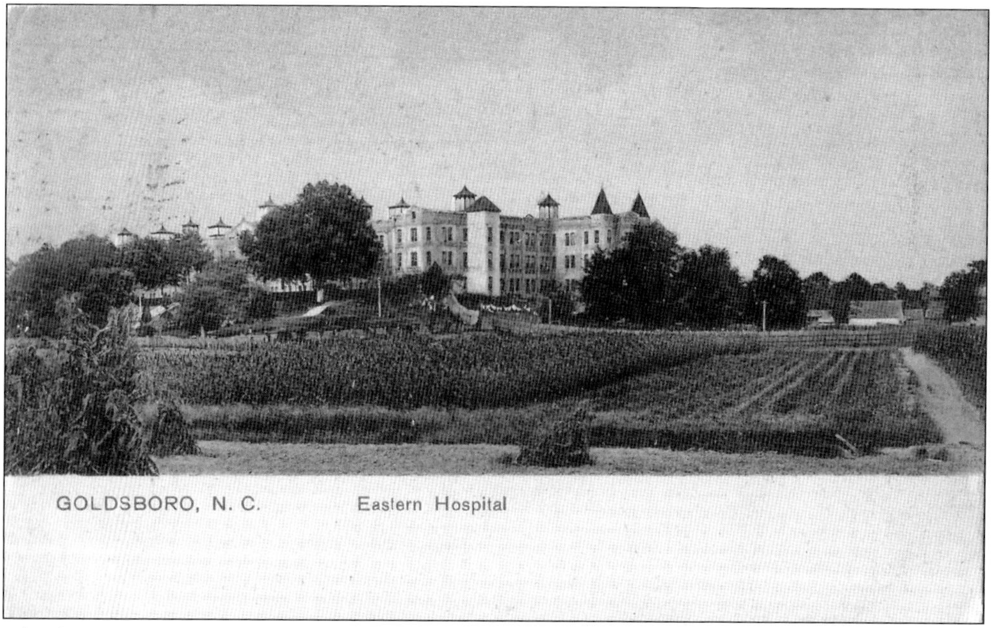

The first patient was admitted to the Asylum for the Colored Insane on August 1, 1880. Gov. Zebulon B. Vance described the site near Goldsboro in Wayne County as ideal because of its "good elevation in a high state of cultivation and central location for the black population."

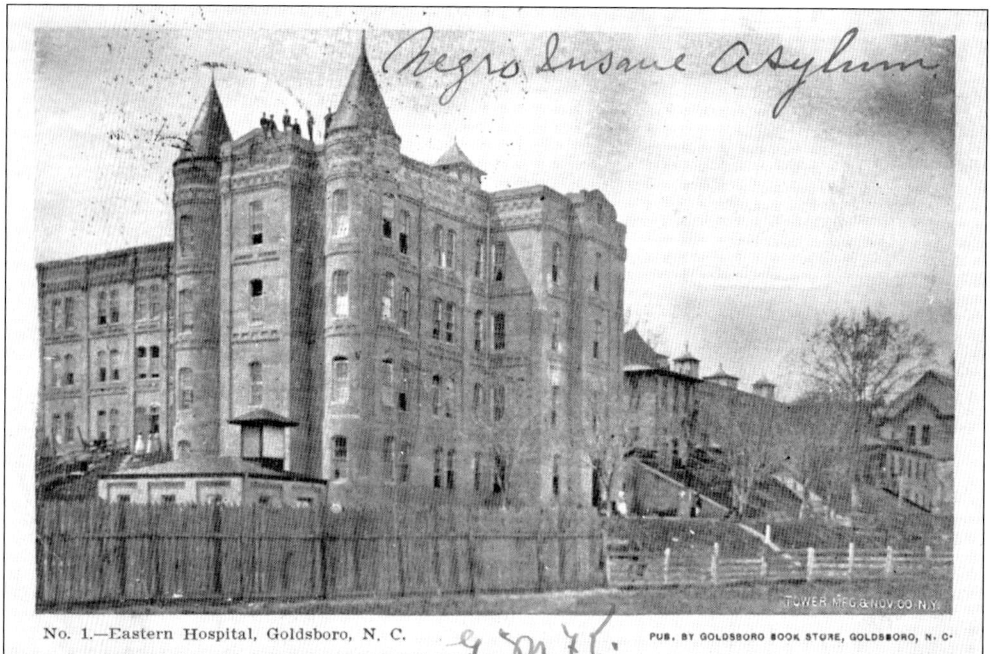

The Eastern Hospital, as identified here, features an early hospital addition aptly referred to as "the castle." Built in the late 1890s, the castle added additional offsets to allow for more windows, following a common architectural design at that time (Moral Treatment, also known as the Kirkbride Plan). The complex was surrounded by fencing, which was supplemented by large ditches. The moat-like appearance further underscored the castle moniker.

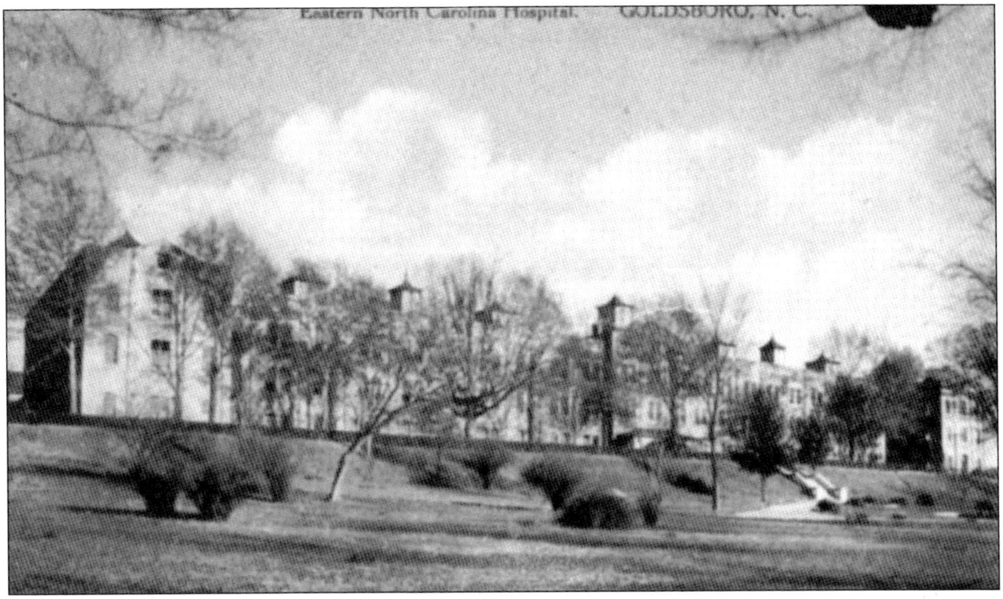

The original asylum endured multiple missions and multiple names. Here, it is identified as the Eastern North Carolina Hospital. By 1923, the hospital was reported to be licensed for 1,066 beds and targeted the "nervous and mental, colored patients," according to the 1923 AMA hospital registry. (Digital NC, presented by the Wayne County Public Library.)

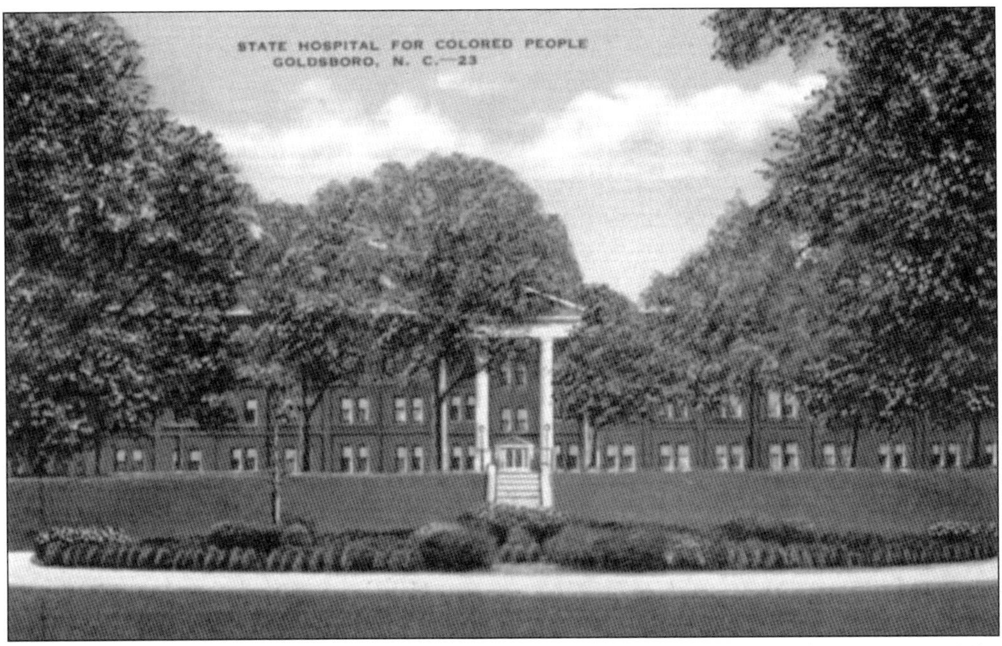

By the late 1940s, the asylum hospital pictured here was referred to as the State Hospital for Colored People. By 1950, the hospital reported 2,770 beds with Dr. I.C. Long as the PIC at that point.

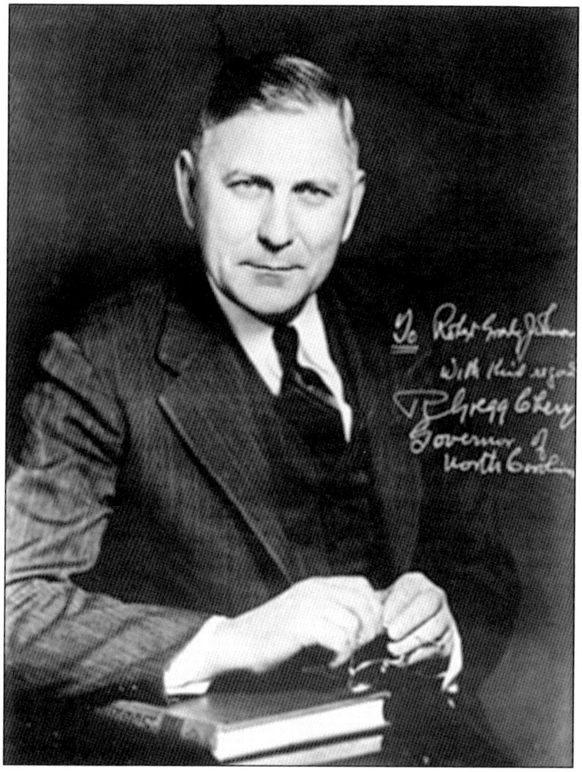

In 1959, Cherry Hospital was renamed in honor of former governor R. Gregg Cherry. He was a devoted and passionate lawmaker who spearheaded the investment into behavioral and mental health in North Carolina. (Photograph no. 132-5. From the Division of Archives and History Photograph Collection, State Archives of North Carolina.)

Approaching the campus from the west, this welcome sign belies what has become more of a series of abandoned buildings. While the campus remains substantial, most of the buildings are now unoccupied and either will be reassigned to another state government agency or demolished.

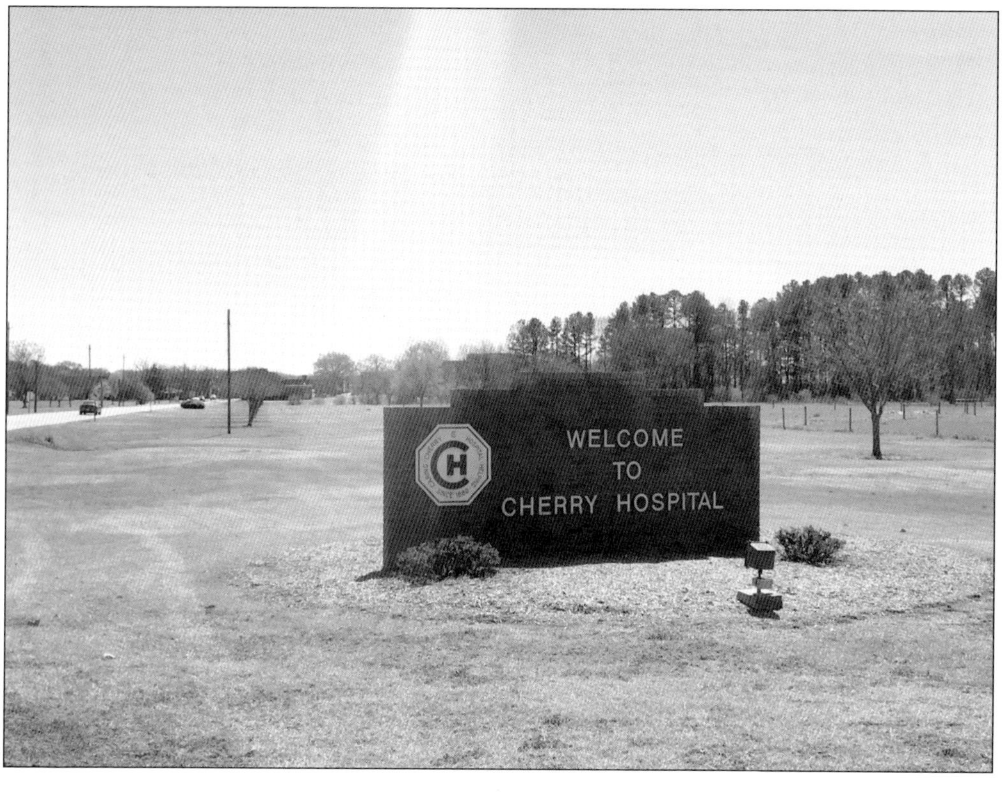

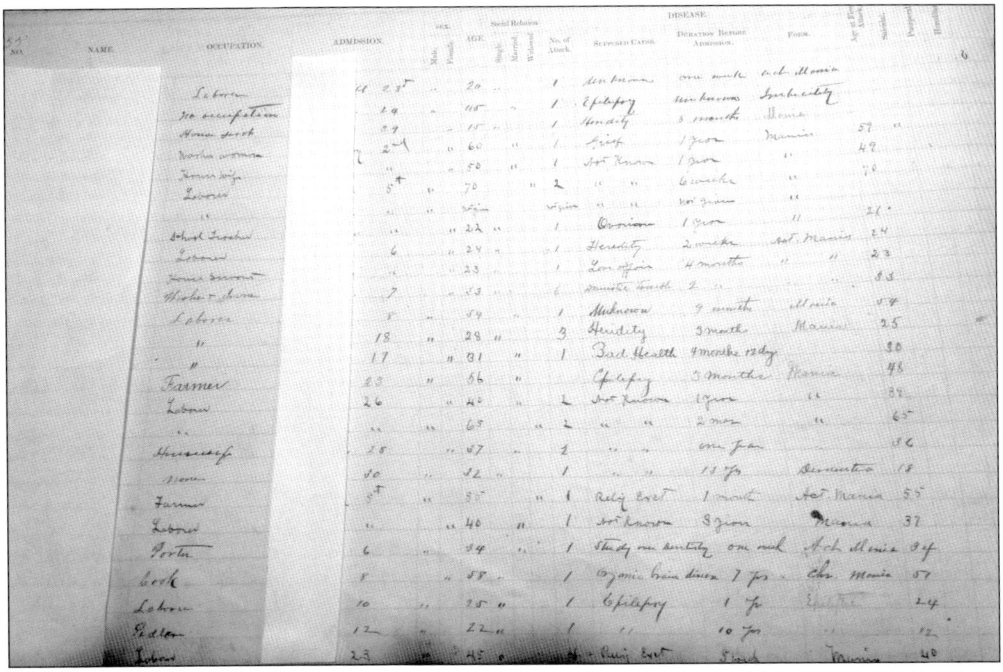

This page from a c. 1905 patient registry at the asylum reveals how this was a place for those whom no one could manage or care for or whom no one wanted. A sample of the admission types from the early 20th century for 26 patients included the following "supposed cause" (conditions): epilepsy (x4), grief, unknown or not known (x10), heredity (x3), love affair, domestic trouble, ovarian, bad health, rely exct (x2), study over dentistry, and organic brain disease. This group of patients ranged in age from 15 to 70. The disease form categories for these 26 patients included imbecility, mania, acute mania, dementia, and epilepsy.

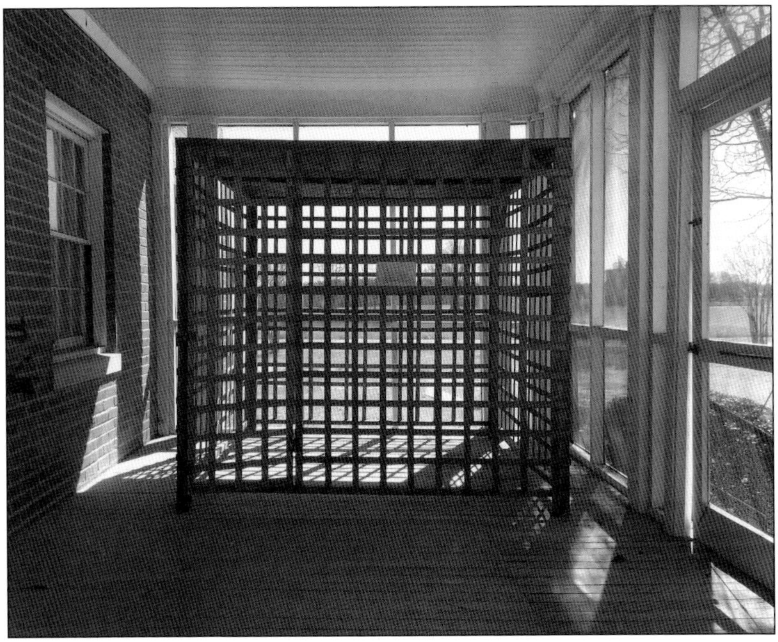

The cage was a means of managing the most difficult and unruly patients. This replica of the cage was on display at the former Cherry Hospital Museum. The museum artifacts are now located at the new hospital complex.

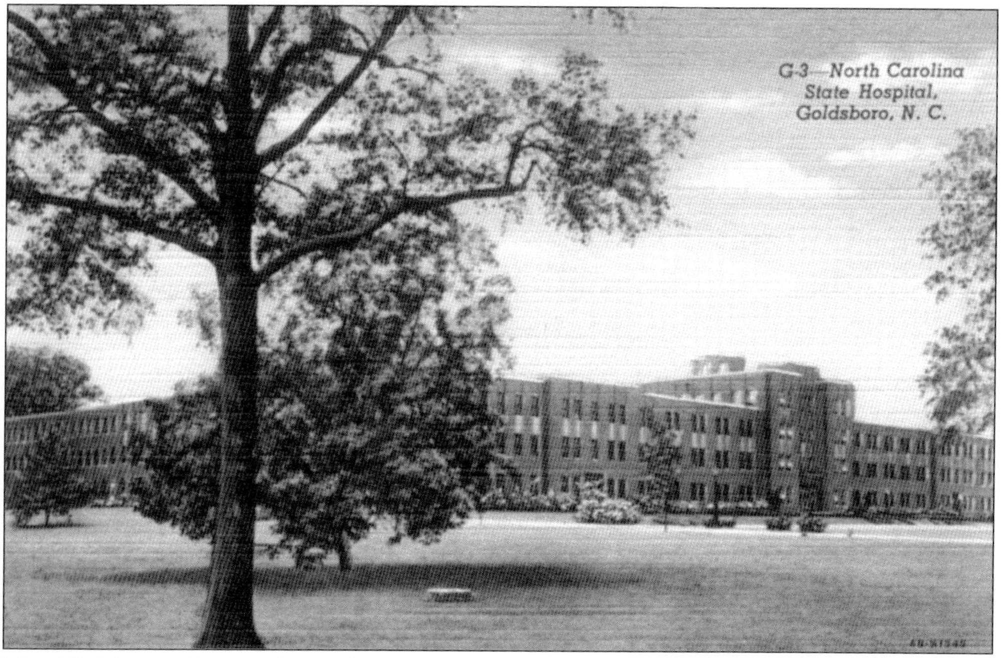

Identified here as the North Carolina State Hospital in the late 1950s, the hospital's mission had included a TB sanatorium, a prison for those deemed mentally unfit to stand trial or criminally insane, and a state hospital for patients with a variety of medical/mental diagnoses. At its largest, the hospital had 4,000-plus patients and more than 6,000 staff but routinely had some 3,000 patients on average in the 1950s and 1960s.

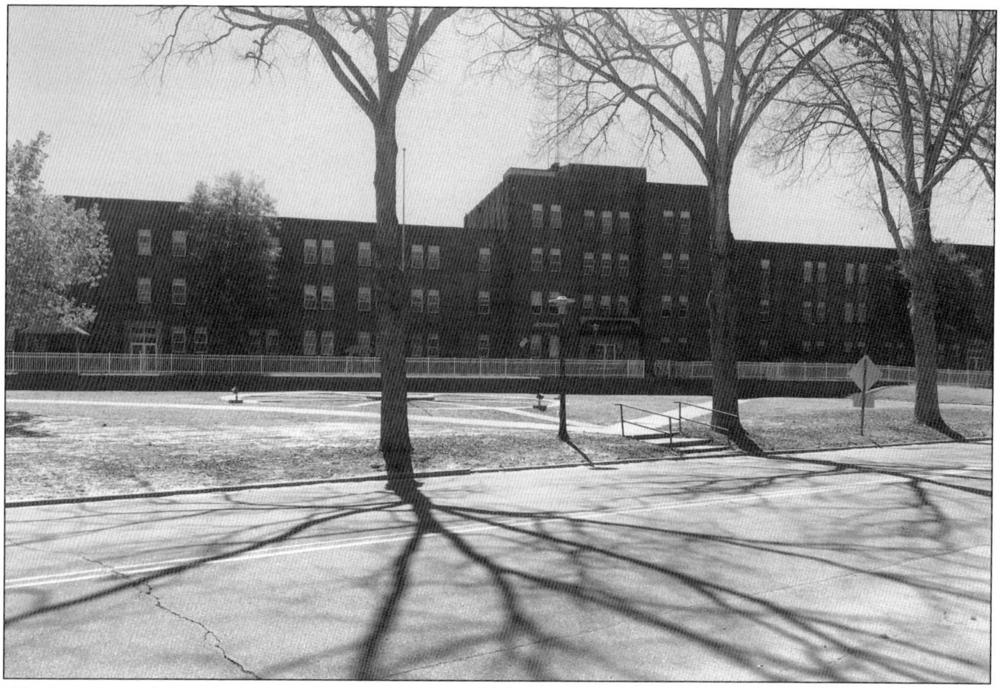

The building shown in the 1950s photograph at the top of this page is mostly unchanged in this 2017 image but awaits a new mission or fate, as it now sits abandoned.

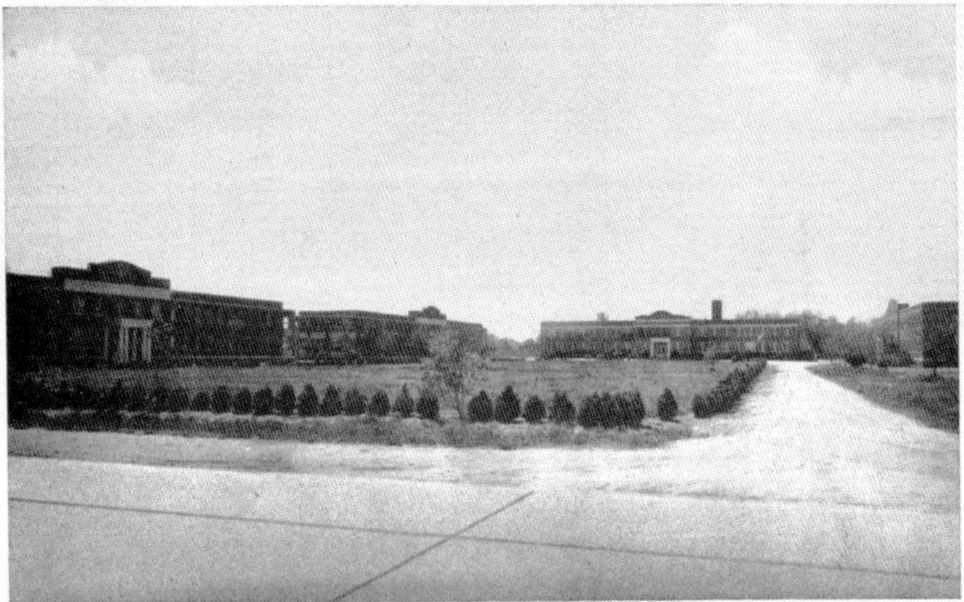

Womens Buildings and N. C. State Hospital, Goldsboro, North Carolina

As the North Carolina State Hospital grew, the need for a separate women's campus became more apparent. While the initial campus included segregated buildings, this approach led to the creation of a new campus constructed on the easternmost side of the campus solely for the female patients. The Women's Campus now is used for the Drug Alcohol Rehabilitation Treatment Program (DART) program and sits just across from the new Cherry Hospital. Pictured above are, from left to right, buildings one, two, three, and four. Building five was not constructed at the time.

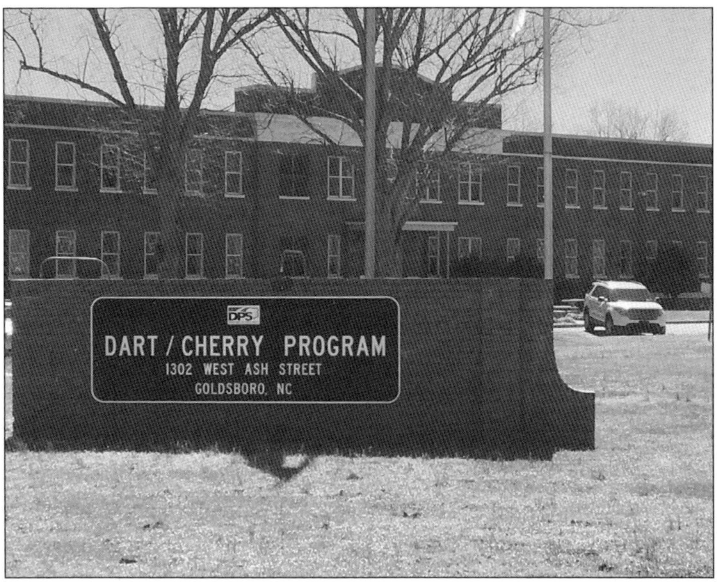

The Drug Alcohol Rehabilitation Treatment Program (DART) is a 300-bed complex across from the new 400-bed Cherry Hospital on West Ash Street in Goldsboro, on the eastern side of the old campus. The DART program now occupies the former Women's Campus of the North Carolina State Hospital. This is building one (and to the right at the edge of the frame is building two).

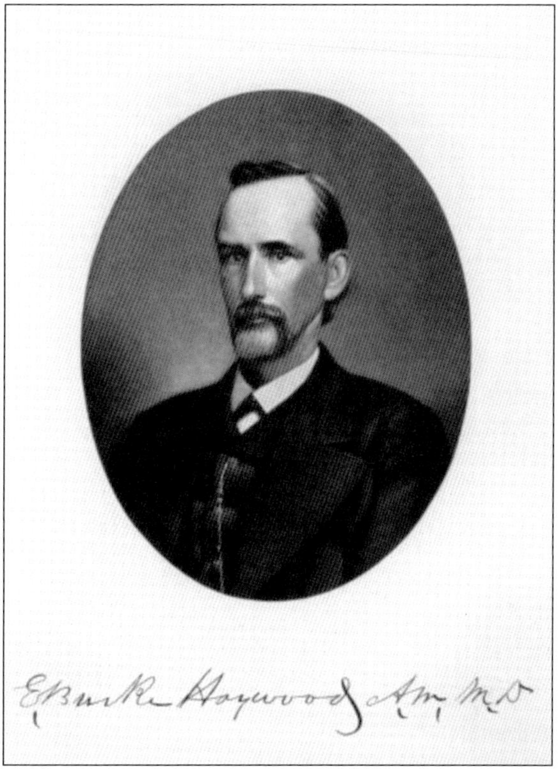

Dr. Edmund Burke Haywood was the chairman of the board of directors for the North Carolina Insane Asylum in the 1870s (which at the time included only the Dorothea Dix Psychiatric Hospital) when he urged the North Carolina General Assembly (NCGA) to develop an asylum for the "blacks of the state" as well as one for Western North Carolina residents. Dr. Haywood had served as the Confederate army surgeon in charge of the Raleigh Confederate Hospitals. Late in the war, he was known for attending to the wounded and ill of both the Union and the Confederacy in the hospitals. (Archive.org.)

The Royster Building was the administration building where many of the patients had remained in the closing days of the old hospital at the center of the campus. It included an emergency department in the rear of the building.

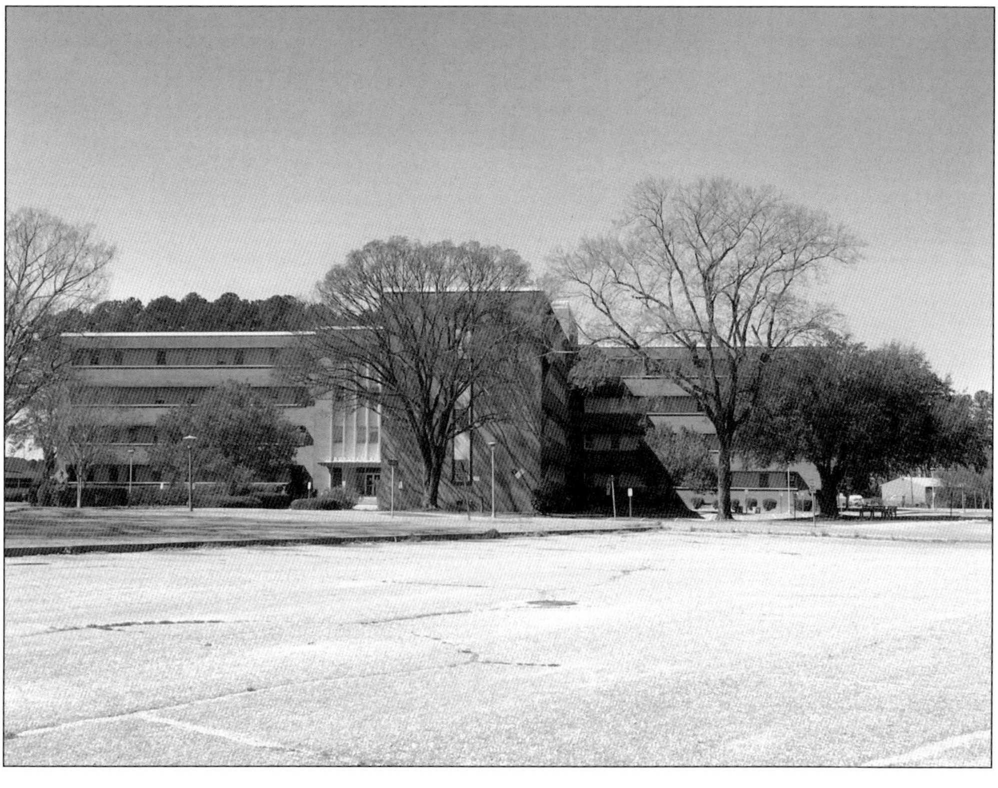

Dr. Ira Hardy (LaGrange) presented a paper at Washington, North Carolina, in December 1910 at the Seaboard Medical Society titled "What It Costs." Dr. Hardy urged his colleagues to consider supporting the establishment of a training school to care for "our Feeble-Minded children." Dr. Hardy's 10-year-old "mentally retarded" daughter died just days later. It became his mission to create a state-sponsored solution to help families with these children. (UNC Digital Library.)

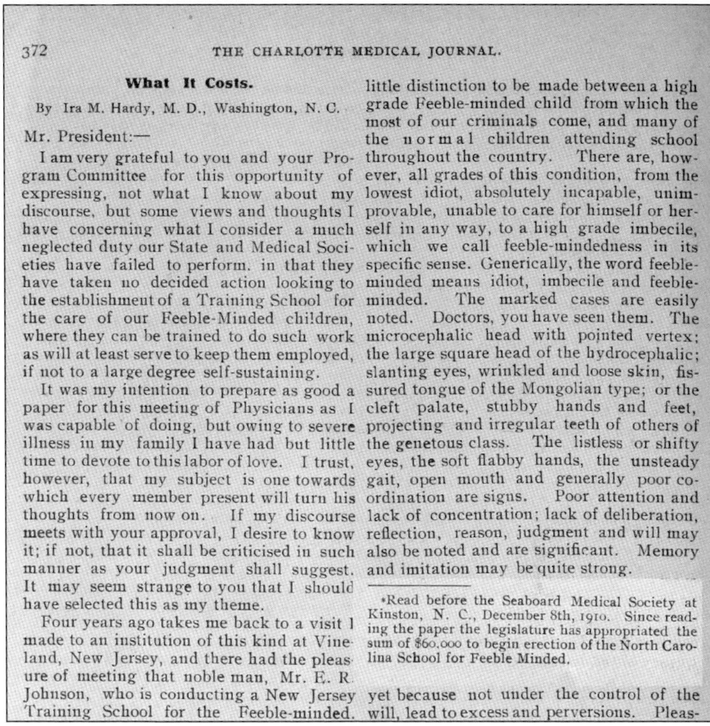

372 THE CHARLOTTE MEDICAL JOURNAL.

What It Costs.

By Ira M. Hardy, M. D., Washington, N. C.

Mr. President:—

I am very grateful to you and your Program Committee for this opportunity of expressing, not what I know about my discourse, but some views and thoughts I have concerning what I consider a much neglected duty our State and Medical Societies have failed to perform, in that they have taken no decided action looking to the establishment of a Training School for the care of our Feeble-Minded children, where they can be trained to do such work as will at least serve to keep them employed, if not to a large degree self-sustaining.

It was my intention to prepare as good a paper for this meeting of Physicians as I was capable of doing, but owing to severe illness in my family I have had but little time to devote to this labor of love. I trust, however, that my subject is one towards which every member present will turn his thoughts from now on. If my discourse meets with your approval, I desire to know it; if not, that it shall be criticised in such manner as your judgment shall suggest. It may seem strange to you that I should have selected this as my theme.

Four years ago takes me back to a visit I made to an institution of this kind at Vineland, New Jersey, and there had the pleasure of meeting that noble man, Mr. E. R. Johnson, who is conducting a New Jersey Training School for the Feeble-minded. little distinction to be made between a high grade Feeble-minded child from which the most of our criminals come, and many of the normal children attending school throughout the country. There are, however, all grades of this condition, from the lowest idiot, absolutely incapable, unimprovable, unable to care for himself or herself in any way, to a high grade imbecile, which we call feeble-mindedness in its specific sense. Generically, the word feeble-minded means idiot, imbecile and feeble-minded. The marked cases are easily noted. Doctors, you have seen them. The microcephalic head with pointed vertex; the large square head of the hydrocephalic; slanting eyes, wrinkled and loose skin, fissured tongue of the Mongolian type; or the cleft palate, stubby hands and feet, projecting and irregular teeth of others of the genetous class. The listless or shifty eyes, the soft flabby hands, the unsteady gait, open mouth and generally poor co-ordination are signs. Poor attention and lack of concentration; lack of deliberation, reflection, reason, judgment and will may also be noted and are significant. Memory and imitation may be quite strong.

*Read before the Seaboard Medical Society at Kinston, N. C., December 8th, 1910. Since reading the paper the legislature has appropriated the sum of $60,000 to begin erection of the North Carolina School for Feeble Minded.

yet because not under the control of the will, lead to excess and perversions. Pleas-

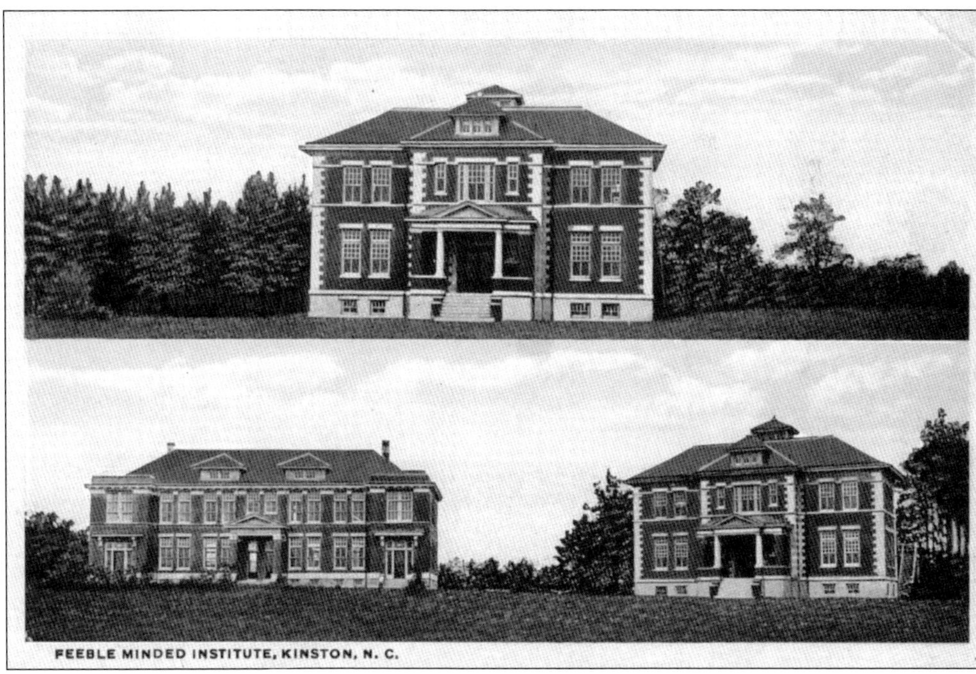

The Feeble-Minded Institute opened at 2415 West Vernon Avenue in Kinston in 1911. The institute served the "backward and mentally defective/deficient." By 1923, the 385-bed facility (27-bed hospital) was renamed for former governor Richard Caswell. By 1956, the facility reported 1,176 beds. Today, the scaled down facility serves a patient population of those with "mental retardation and developmental disabilities."

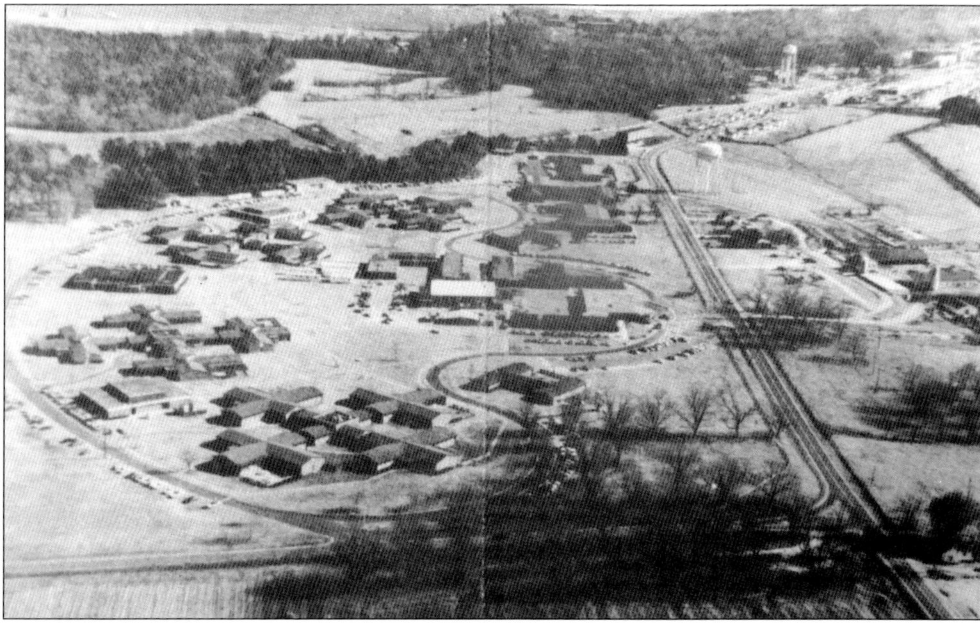

In 1957, the Goldsboro Training School opened as the nation's first school dedicated to the treatment of the "colored, feeble-minded" patients, instead of sending them to an asylum. The Goldsboro Training School included a large campus of buildings for education and teaching basic trades. It also included a large farm area where residents raised crops to support the school. (Wayne County Public Library.)

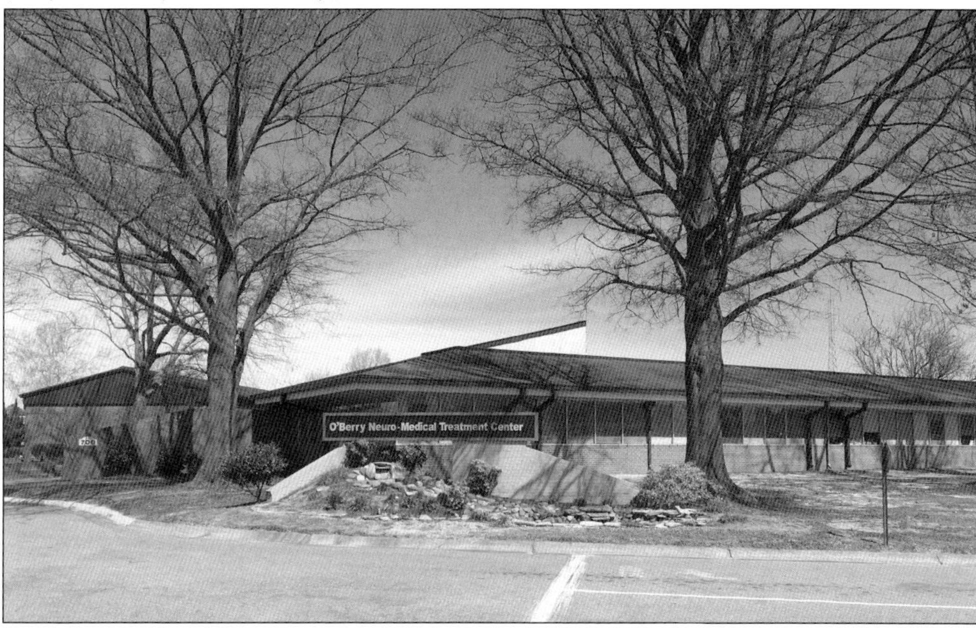

Today, the Goldsboro Training School is known as the O'Berry Neuro-Medical Treatment Center. The campus of more than a dozen buildings borders the Cherry Hospital campus. The O'Berry Neuro-Medical Treatment Center became a long-term care hospital before transitioning to a skilled nursing facility serving more than 400 patients considered intellectually disabled with long-term neurological needs.

Two

Sanatoriums

The typical sanatorium was built and owned by one or two physicians and included a residence for the physician and his family. The physician (or physicians) who lived in the building cared for patients along with a staff of aides and nurses. These facilities emerged in the late 19th century and became popular in the first half of the 20th century. Multiple private sanatoriums could be found across Eastern North Carolina by 1930.

The state sanatoriums were more likely to be built for specialty needs or specific chronic health conditions. This primarily included tuberculosis (TB) and mostly accommodated patients of limited financial support. By 1800, it was believed that approximately 15 percent of the world's population had died because of TB (also referred to as consumption, Pott's Disease, or the white plague). By the early 1900s, TB was the leading cause of death for North Carolinians. At their peak, many of the state sanatoriums were massive, caring for thousands of patients suffering from TB and other chronic diseases.

The factors that led to the eventual closure of many smaller sanatoriums across the state included the change in health of the physician/owner, competition for limited staff with other sanatoriums, and the emergence of the general hospital. However, the final blow to the sanatorium followed the discovery of the antibiotic that changed the healing process from months to days. By the early 1950s, sanatoriums were closing or had transformed into general hospitals.

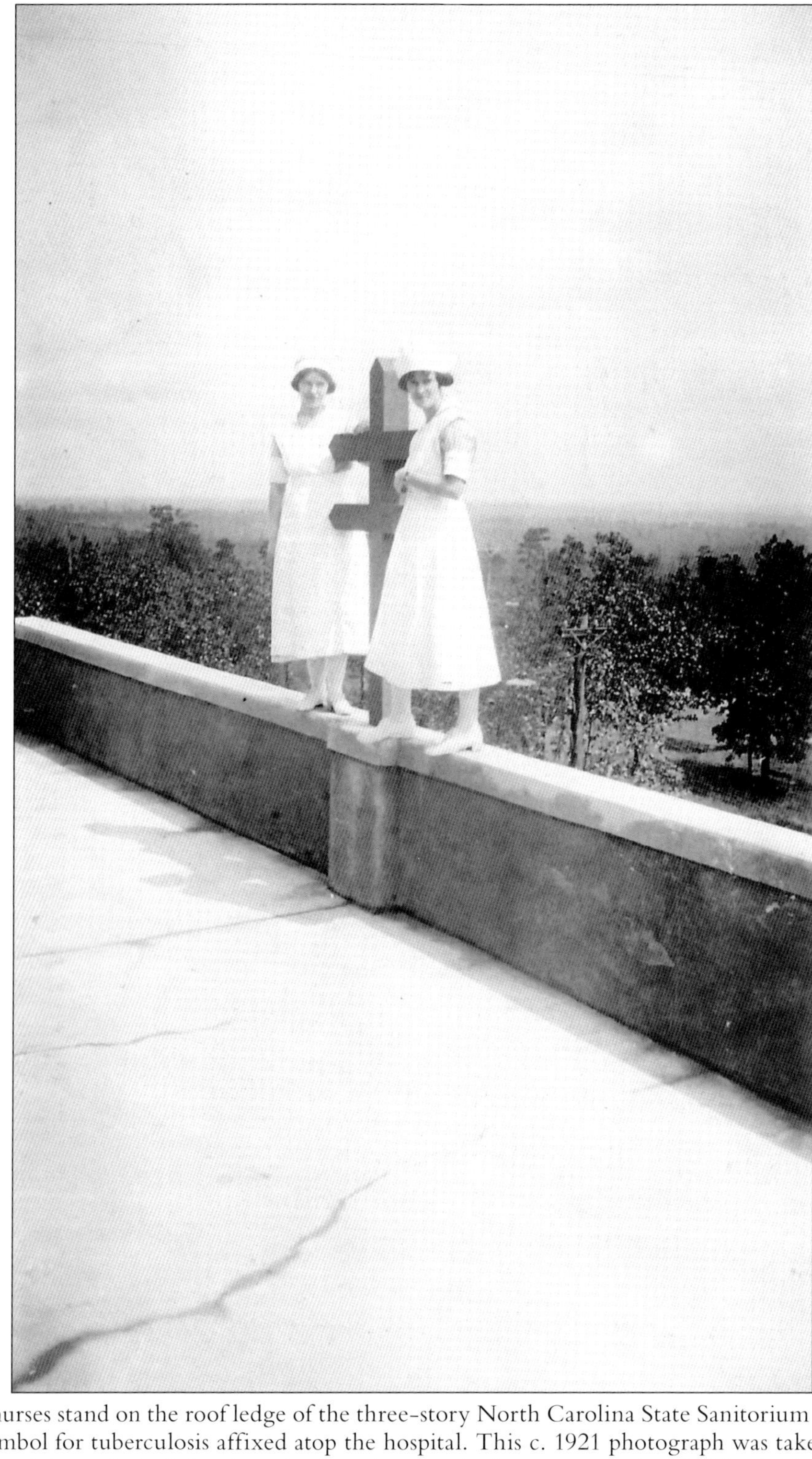

Two nurses stand on the roof ledge of the three-story North Carolina State Sanitorium next to the symbol for tuberculosis affixed atop the hospital. This c. 1921 photograph was taken from the top of the main building for what later became the largest sanatorium in North Carolina.

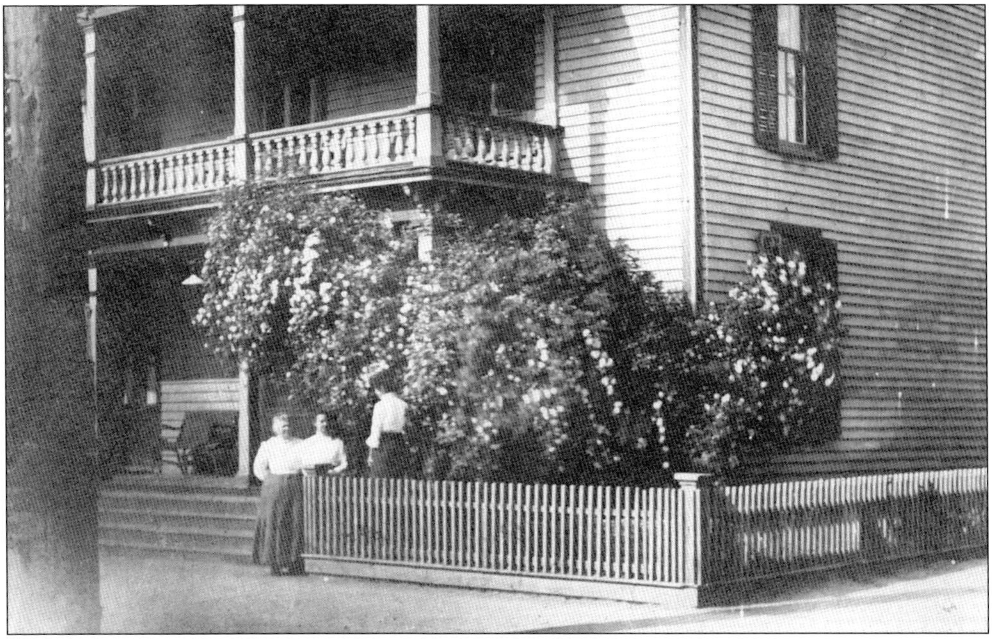

Dr. H.O. Hyatt's Sanatorium for the Disease of the Eye and General Surgery was established in 1890 as a private hospital in Kinston (Lenoir County). In 1912, it was a 10-bed facility. By 1915, the building (pictured here) was identified as the Hyatt Boarding House. (Durwood Barbour Collection, Wilson Library, UNC-Chapel Hill.)

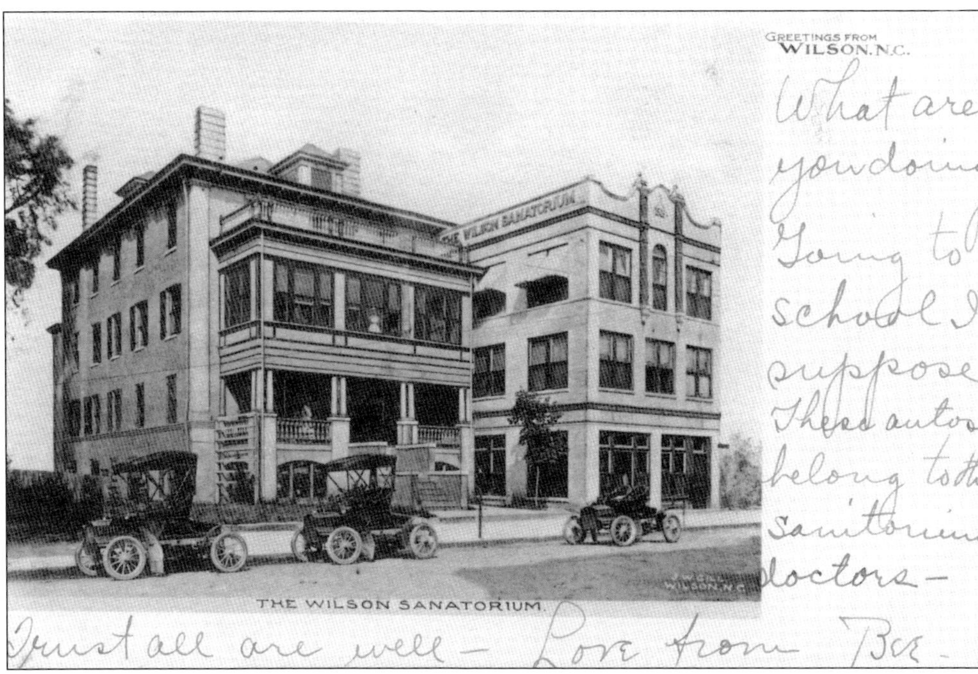
GREETINGS FROM
WILSON, N.C.
What are you doing Going to school I suppose These autos belong to the sanitorium doctors -
THE WILSON SANATORIUM
THE WILSON SANATORIUM.
Trust all are well - Love from Bee.

The Wilson Sanitorium was located at 216–218 East Nash Street. Established in 1895 as a 25-bed hospital, the PIC was Dr. E.T. Dickinson in 1923. (Durwood Barbour Collection, Wilson Library, UNC-Chapel Hill.)

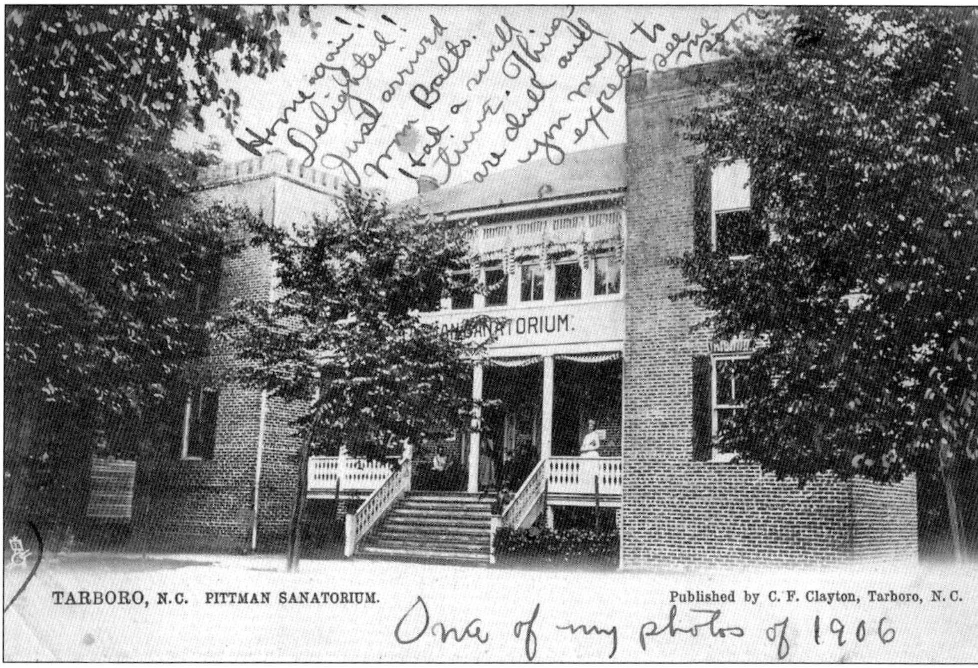

In 1901, the 20-bed Pittman Sanatorium was established as a public hospital at 305 St. Andrews Street in Tarboro (Edgecombe County). In 1906, the physicians who opened the hospital included L.L. Staton, J.M. Barker, S.N. Harrell, W.J. Thigpen, and J.J. Phillips. By 1912, the 25-bed hospital was led by Dr. M.T. Shackleford (PIC). The sanatorium became Edgecombe General in 1916.

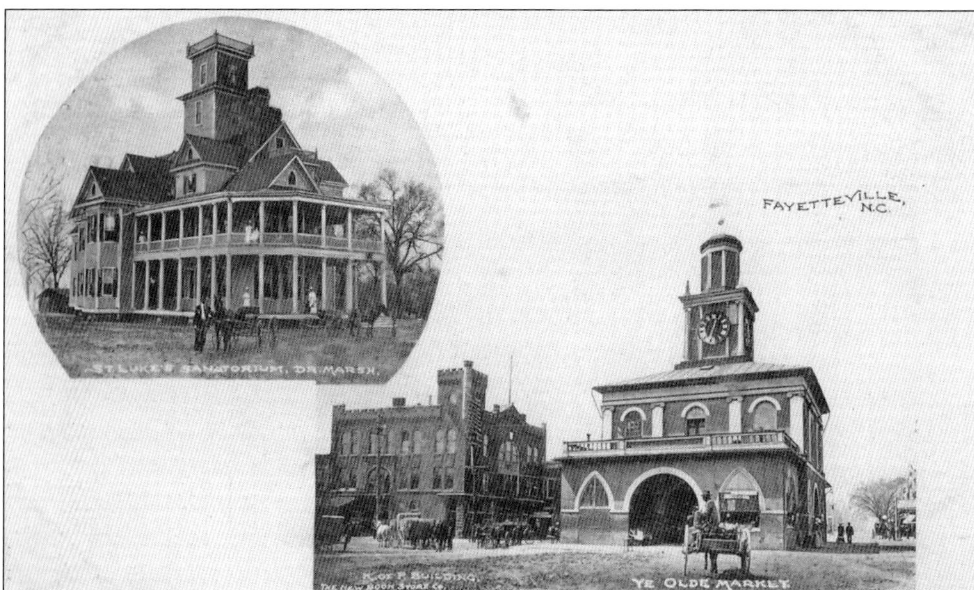

St. Luke's Sanatorium opened in 1905 in Fayetteville. Dr. J.H. Marsh, who had partnered with Dr. Highsmith when the Highsmith Marsh Sanitorium first opened in Fayetteville, was the PIC. St. Luke's Sanatorium would later become known as St. Luke's Hospital and Dr. Marsh's Sanatorium. By 1916, the sanatorium was no longer listed in the AMA hospital registry.

The Martha Moore Sanatorium was converted to a 20-bed hospital in Elm City (Wilson County) in 1906. By 1914, it was no longer listed as a hospital. The building lived out its life as a private residence before being demolished in the 1970s. The original name of the town was Toisnot, but locally it was referred to as Elm City before the official change occurred in 1913. (Durwood Barbour Collection, Wilson Library, UNC-Chapel Hill.)

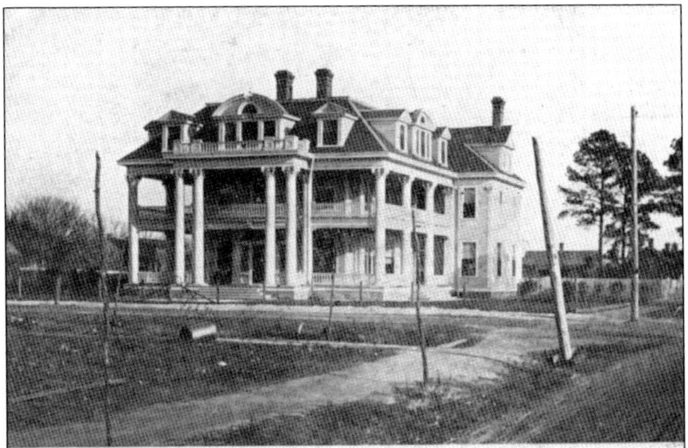

Martha Moore Sanatorium, Elm City, N. C. Pub. by Barnes & Winstead.

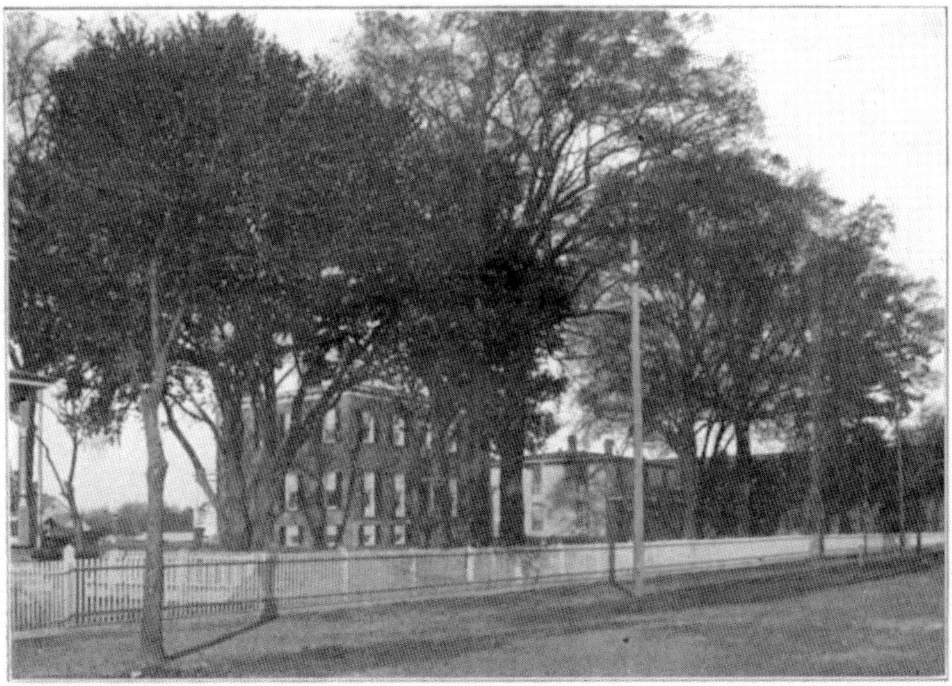

Stewart's Sanitorium, New Bern, N. C.

Owned by John Washington Stewart (who also owned the Hazelton Hotel), the Stewart Sanatorium was located northwest of Cedar Grove Cemetery in New Bern. The sanatorium opened July 15, 1908, and operated as a public hospital. By 1912, the 21-bed hospital was led by Maybelle Corington, superintendent. The building was destroyed in the great New Bern fire (1922). (New Bern Public Library.)

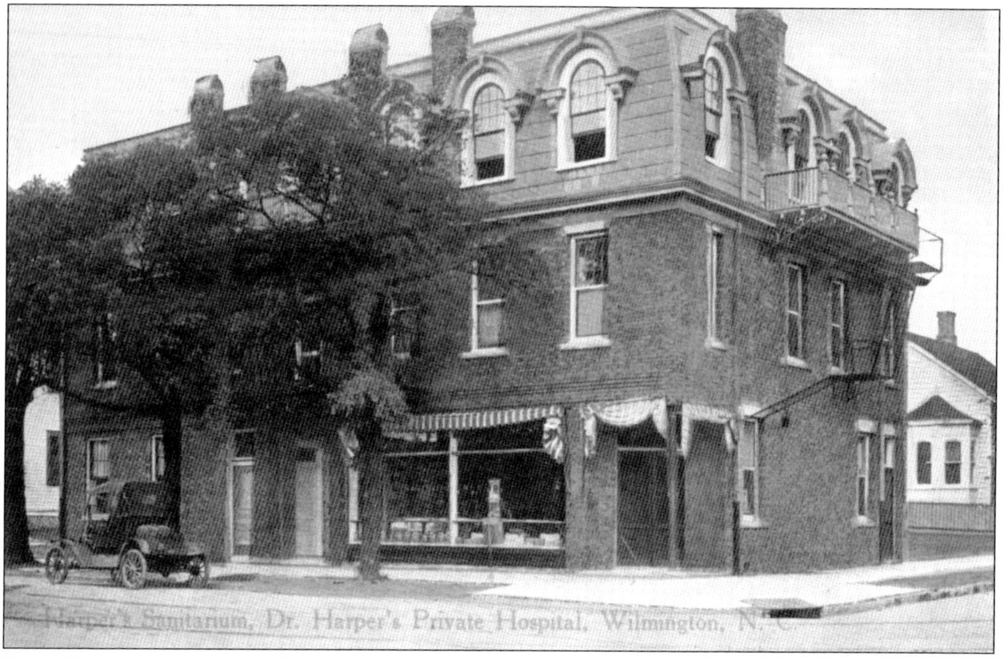

Dr. Charles Harper was the Wilmington superintendent of health until 1909. In 1910, he opened Harper's Sanitarium, on Front and Castle Streets. In 1913, Dr. Harper was appointed district assistant surgeon by the Seaboard Air Line Railway. While the exact closure date was not identified, the sanitarium was no longer listed as a hospital in 1921. (Durwood Barbour Collection, Wilson Library, UNC-Chapel Hill.)

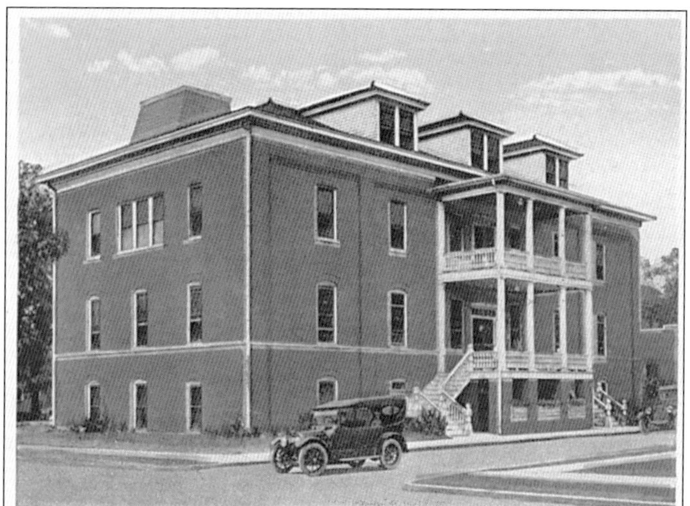

ROCKY MOUNT SANITARIUM.

The Rocky Mount Sanitarium opened in 1913. Three doctors started the sanitarium: L.W. Kornegay, John L. Lane, and Walter Staley. It operated as a 30-bed general hospital and included a nurse training program as well as an ambulance service. In 1920, the hospital was enlarged and remodeled. In 1922, the hospital was briefly owned by the Franciscan Order of Nuns but was sold back to Dr. Kornegay by year's end.

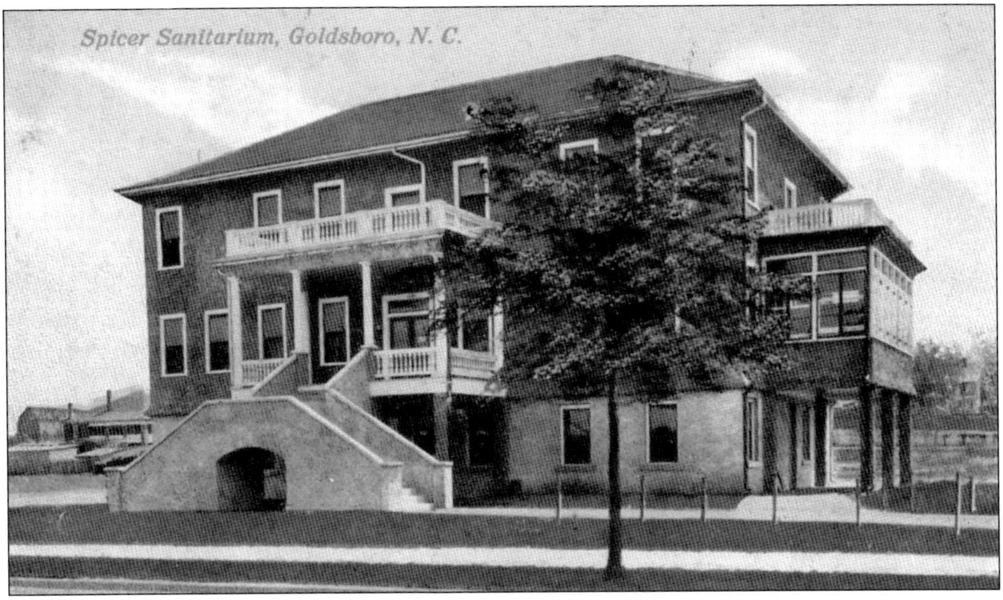

Dr. William Spicer's 25-bed sanitarium (also printed as sanatorium) was established in 1914. The sanitarium was the only approved Goldsboro hospital for nurse training in 1931. The Spicer Sanitarium, later operated by the Spicer brothers (doctors), closed in 1944 after the death of one brother and the poor health of the other. The sanitarium once stood on West Ash Street, near the train station.

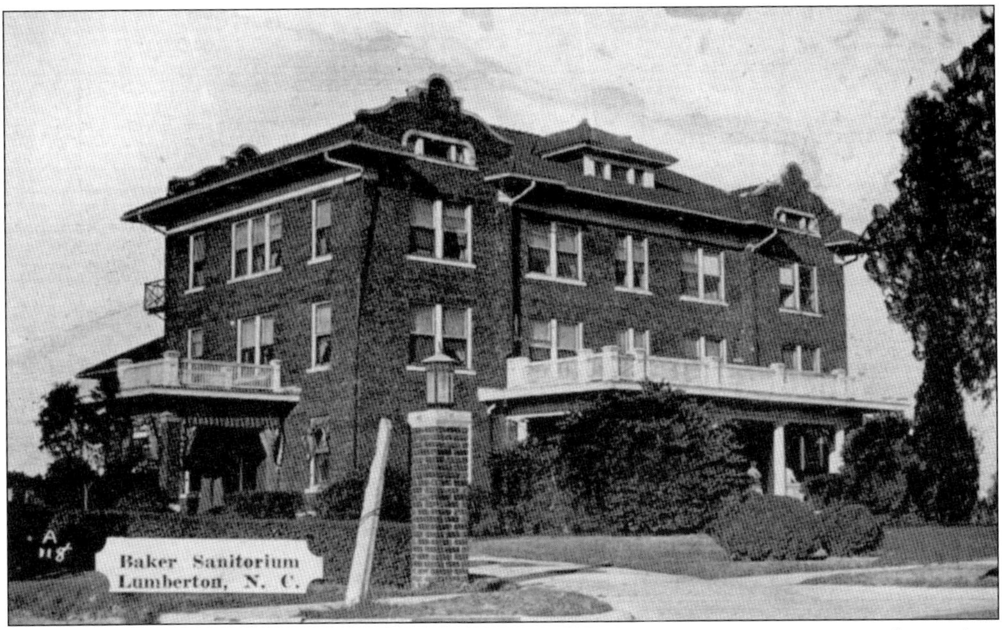

Dr. Horace M. Baker opened the Baker Sanitorium in February 1921. It was located at Fourteenth and Chestnut Streets in Lumberton. By 1923, the 40-bed sanitorium was staffed by Dr. Baker, Dr. Russell S. Beam, Dr. C.V. West, and Dr. H.T. Pope. Baker Sanitorium later merged with Thompson Hospital after Dr. Thomas Clarence Johnson's 1945 death to form Baker-Thompson Memorial Hospital. The hospital was replaced in 1953 by Robeson County Memorial Hospital.

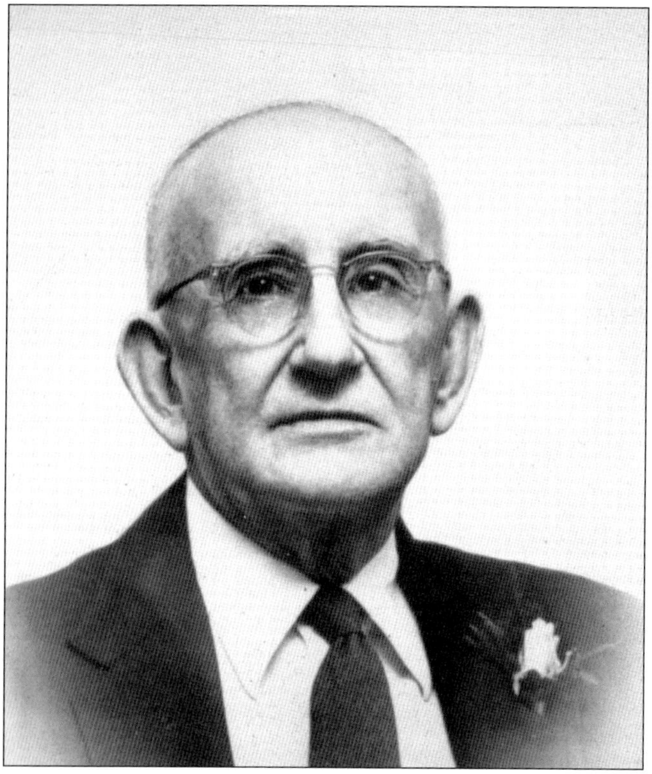

Dr. John C. Wessell (1877–1960) was a Wilmington-area physician who dedicated much of his life to public health and combating the white plague (also known as tuberculosis). The Tuberculosis Hospital came to be known as the Wessell Sanitorium. (New Hanover County Public Library.)

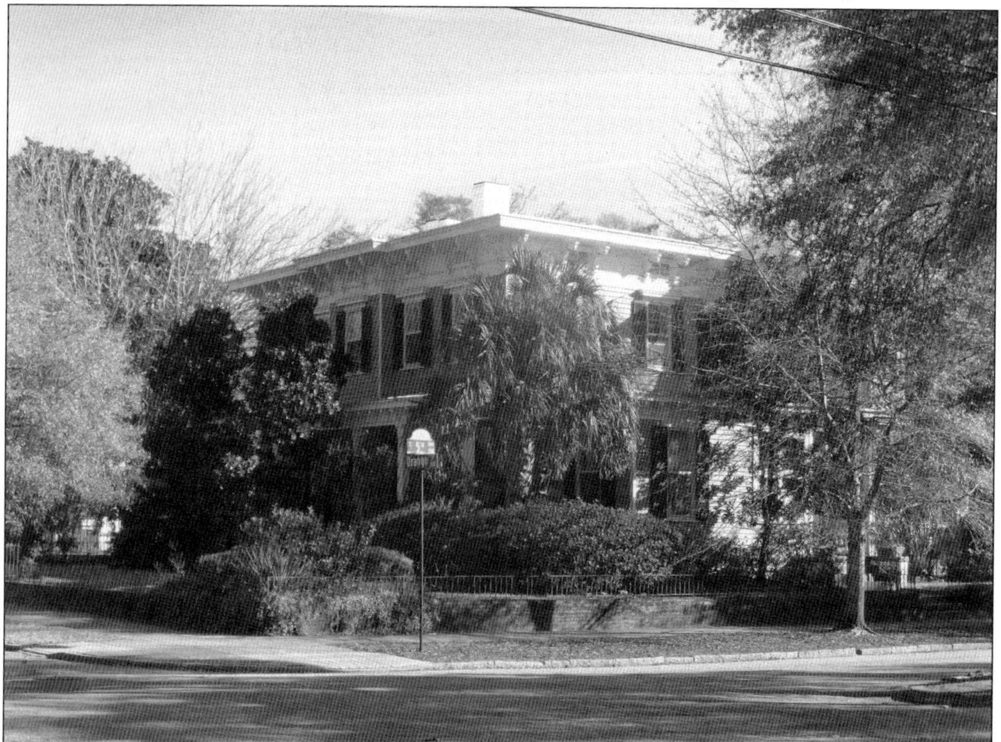

St. John's Sanitorium opened as a 22-bed general hospital in 1919 in Wilmington. It was located at 504 Orange Street, with Dr. John F. Miller as the PIC. Today, the property is historically restored and used as a multifamily property with apartments and a private residence (Woodbury Hoggard House).

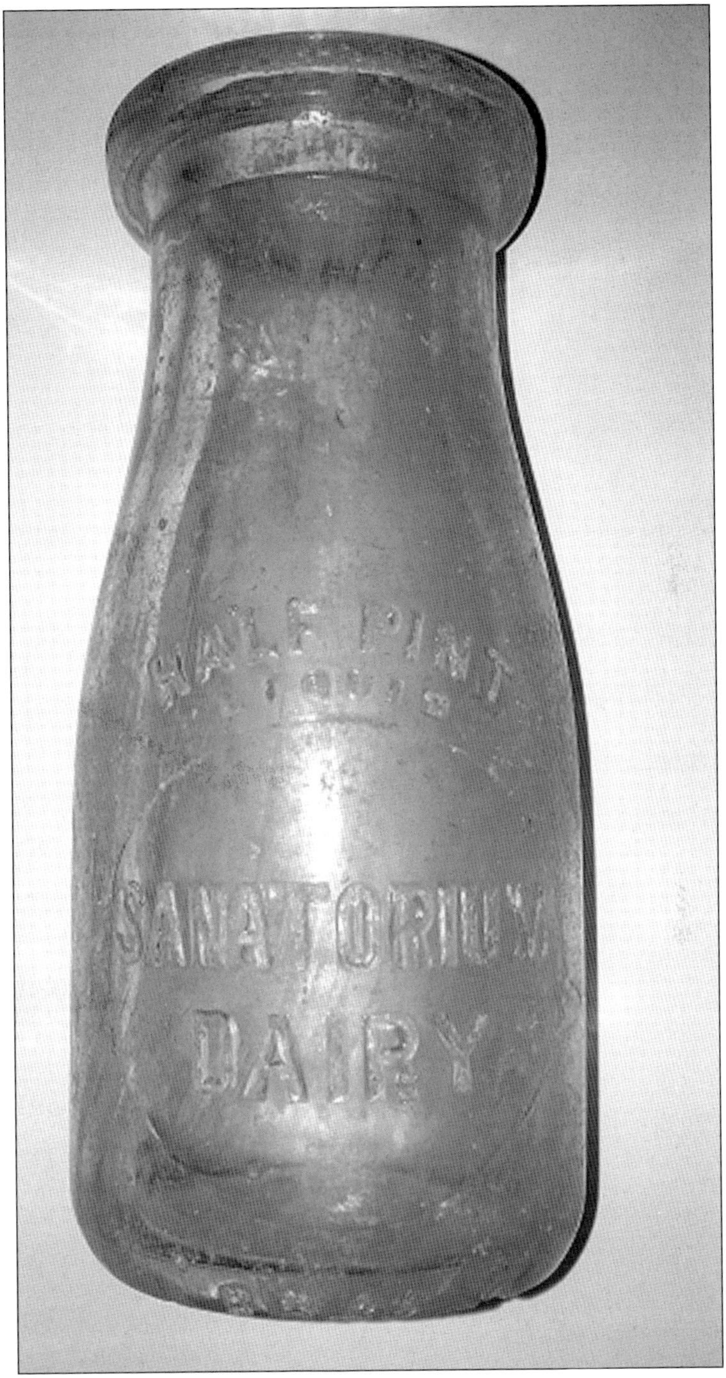

Pictured here is a North Carolina Sanatorium dairy bottle. By the 1940s, the state sanatoriums and asylums typically sold their excess products to support the mission. The more than 2,000 acres were managed by staff and able-bodied patients to feed people on the campus. They had everything from fruit trees and sugar cane to wheat and a wide variety of vegetables. The animals used to feed the patients included pigs, turkeys, chickens, and cows for both milk and beef.

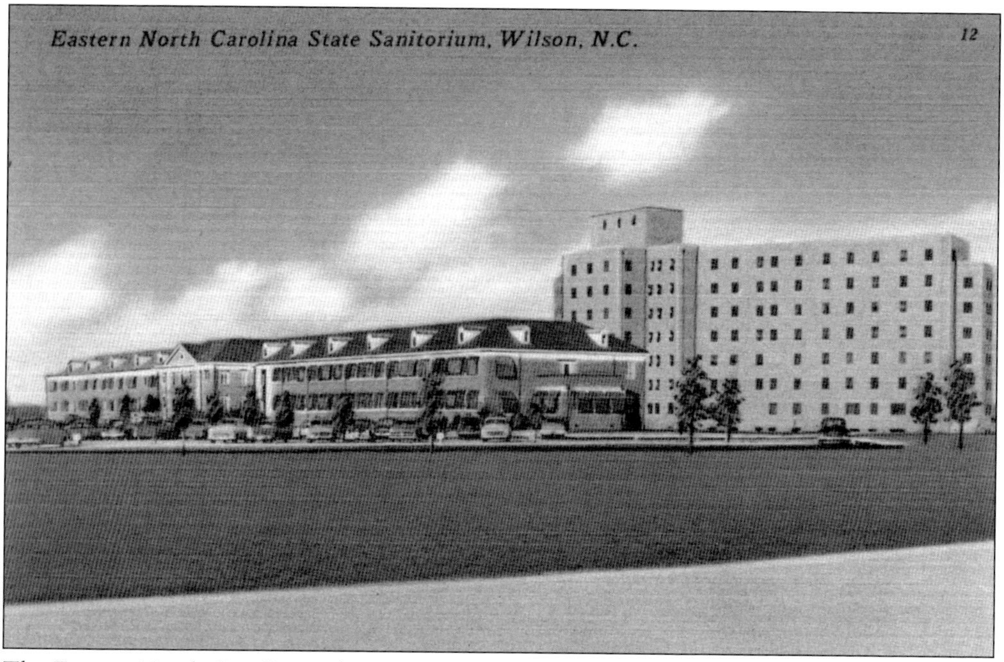

The Eastern North Carolina Tuberculosis Sanitorium opened in 1942 in Wilson. The facility has undergone several missions and today serves patients with mental disabilities. Now known as the Longleaf Neuro-Medical Treatment Center, it is a sister facility to the O'Berry Center. (Durwood Barbour Collection, Wilson Library, UNC-Chapel Hill.)

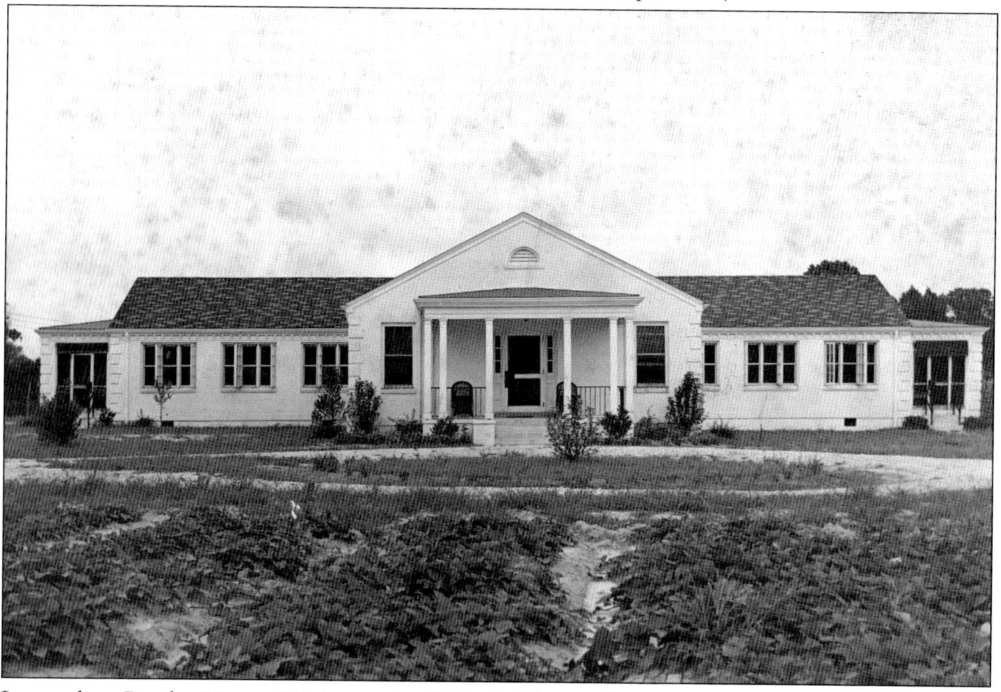

Located on Rocky Mount Highway, the 27-bed Edgecombe County Tuberculosis Sanatorium was established in 1920 in Tarboro (Edgecombe County). In 1956, Dr. William B. Hooks was the PIC. (Digital NC, Edgecombe County Memorial Library.)

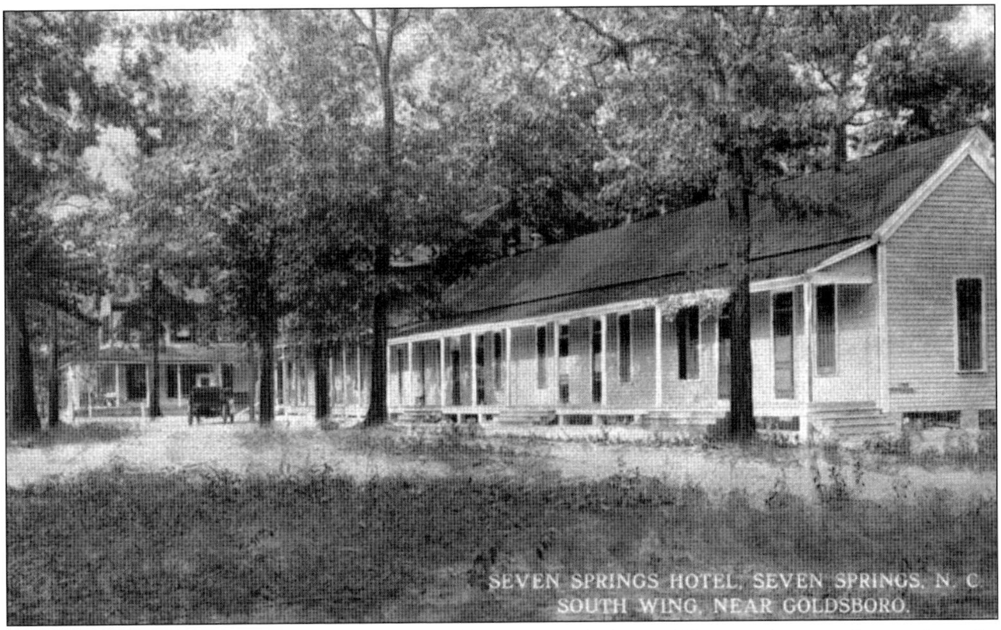
SEVEN SPRINGS HOTEL, SEVEN SPRINGS, N. C.
SOUTH WING, NEAR GOLDSBORO.

The south wing of the Seven Springs Hotel is pictured above. The caption on the card reads, "Since nature has a remedy for all of our ills, Enlightened people have stopped taking pills. Very many that once suffered aches and pains, earnestly drink nature's remedy and are well again. No reason why you should suffer more, Since the remedy for all ills is here in store. Peace to the troubled soul you'll find, Rest for the overburdened mind. In fact, a surcease from all care, God's remedy for all ill that man brings, Source of health—Seven Springs." (Durwood Barbour Collection, Wilson Library, UNC-Chapel Hill.)

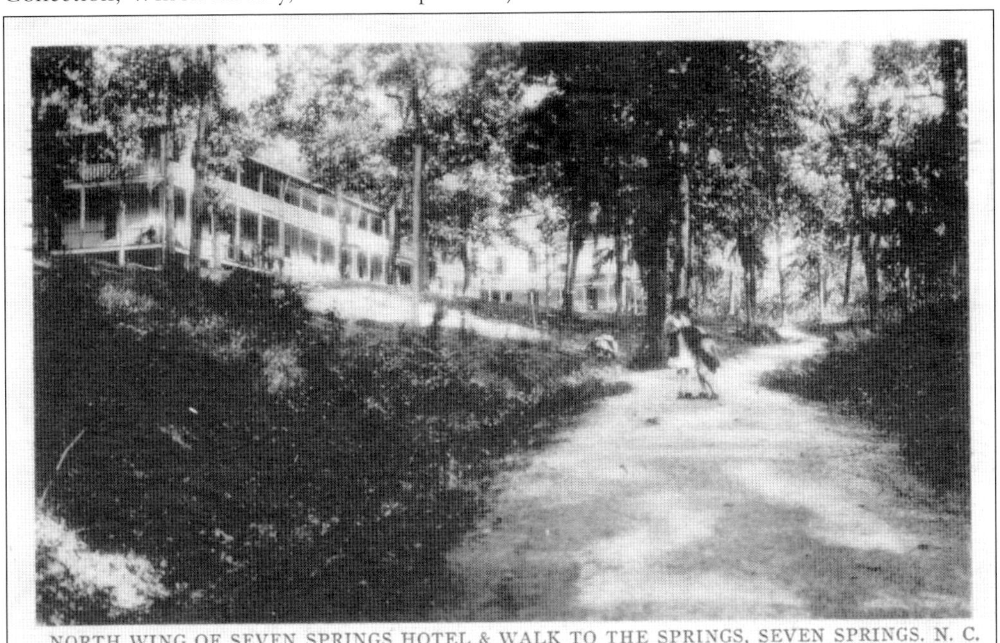
NORTH WING OF SEVEN SPRINGS HOTEL & WALK TO THE SPRINGS, SEVEN SPRINGS. N. C.

The Seven Springs Hotel in Wayne County was a classic example of a resort also commonly referred to as a sanitarium.

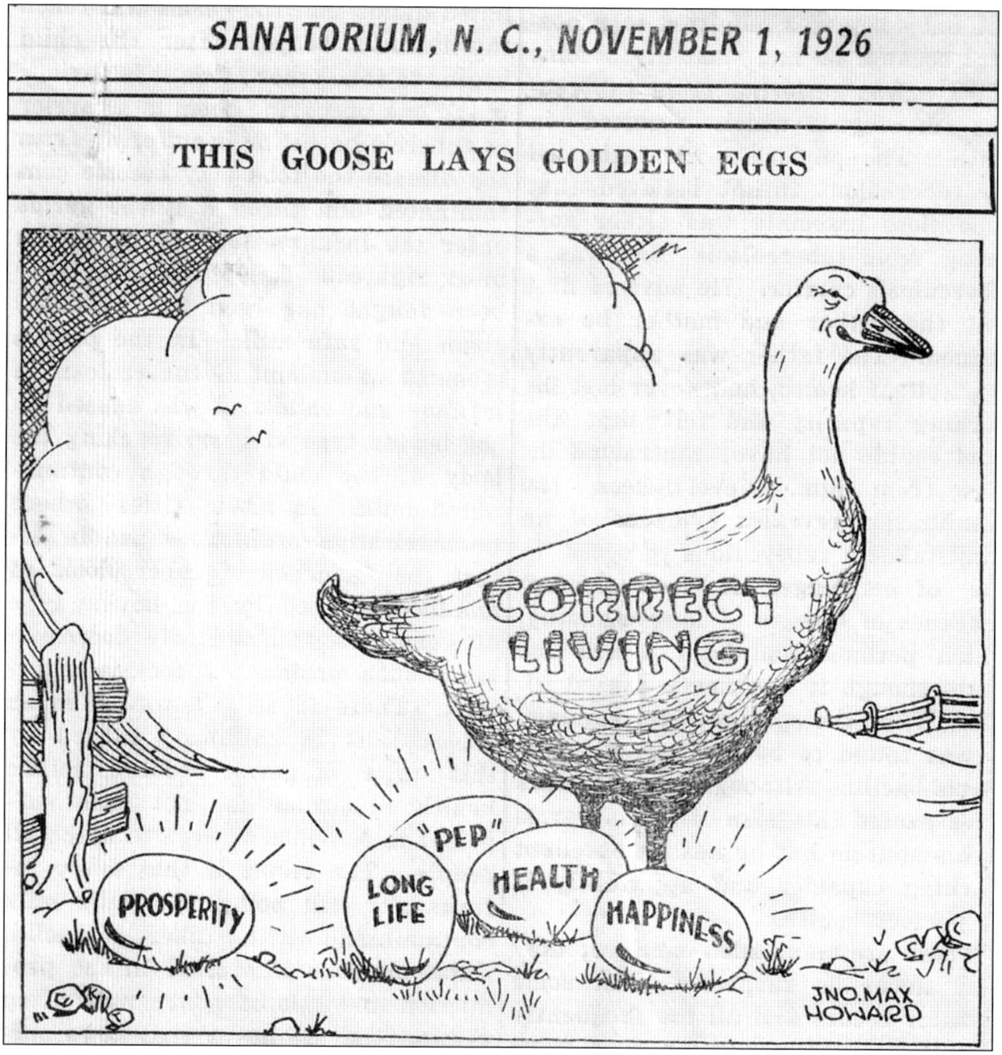

This image is a clipping from a newspaper, the *Sanatorium*, and denotes a message befitting of what the sanatorium instilled, that "correct living" leads to a long and healthy life. The town and post office were also called Sanatorium and located in what was, at the time, western Cumberland County. What remains of the state sanatorium complex on Highway 211 is now in an area known as McCain, in Hoke County, just east of Aberdeen.

Three

Marine, Port, and Railroad Hospitals

The early 19th century relied heavily on shipping as a means of trading European goods for American raw materials in the United States. The US Marine Hospital Service (predecessor to the US Public Health Service) was created by Congress in 1798 to provide medical care for sick and disabled mariners. Paid for by taxing sailors 20¢ per month, it became the first US medical insurance program.

By 1835, Ocracoke and Wilmington were North Carolina's busiest ports. Portsmouth Village became the duty station for Port Ocracoke as the ships arrived at the inlet between the villages. By 1860, two of the 27 US Marine Hospitals, located at ocean or river ports, included Portsmouth and Wilmington.

A hurricane struck the Portsmouth/Ocracoke area on September 6, 1846, pushing substantial storm surge (water) into Pamlico Sound. By the next morning, the eye of the hurricane moved ashore, and counterclockwise winds that were once driving water into the sound, now furiously pushed it back out to sea. The long peninsula, which once stretched from Kitty Hawk to Ocracoke Village, was breached south of Manteo as well as near Hatteras Village. The *Oregon* was the first ship to sail through the newly created inlet near Manteo. Charted as the Oregon Inlet, this new path forever changed regional shipping routes.

Quarantine for sailors exhibiting signs and symptoms of illnesses could be traced to the 1751 Pilotage Act. Wilmington witnessed significant outbreaks of yellow fever, one in the early 1820s and another in 1862. The 1862 outbreak, blamed on sick sailors from a blockade runner, killed over 600. After the war, additional quarantine camps (or lazarettos) were built at various ports by both state and federal authorities. Some were built on stilts in the water to allow ships to dock and offload sickened sailors without them ever entering the city.

Shipping and rail services grew as the ports became larger and rail became the principal means of moving people and goods across the state. As small sanatoriums gave way to municipal hospitals, these buildings were constructed either close to the water or rail for ease of movement. The growth of the railroads also led to the creation of "railroad employee only" hospitals, typically built at a major hub.

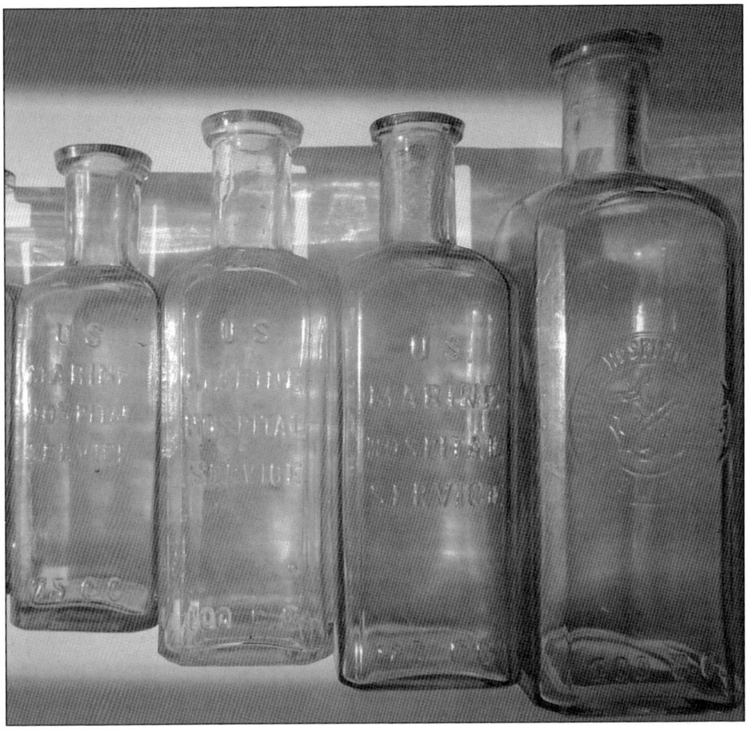

In 1828, a small house in Portsmouth Village was leased for use as a US Marine Hospital (Carteret County) with Dr. John Potts serving as the PIC. This was the first hospital in North Carolina. In 1842, Congress appropriated $8,500 to build a permanent hospital there. At its peak, the 300-bed hospital included 18 physicians and medical lectures for students. These bottles are relics from a US Marine Hospital.

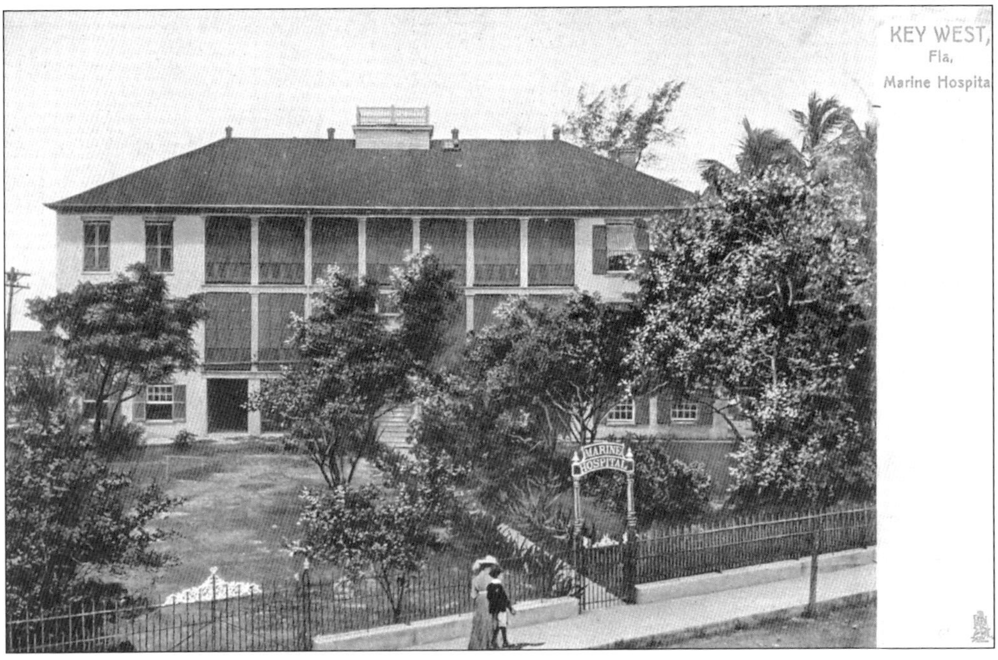

The new US Marine Hospital at Portsmouth Village opened in 1847. There is no known photograph of the Portsmouth hospital. However, architecturally, it shared a Robert Mills design with the Key West US Marine Hospital built in 1844 (and pictured here). The Portsmouth hospital deviated from the Key West hospital by including a fireplace in each room and was less elevated.

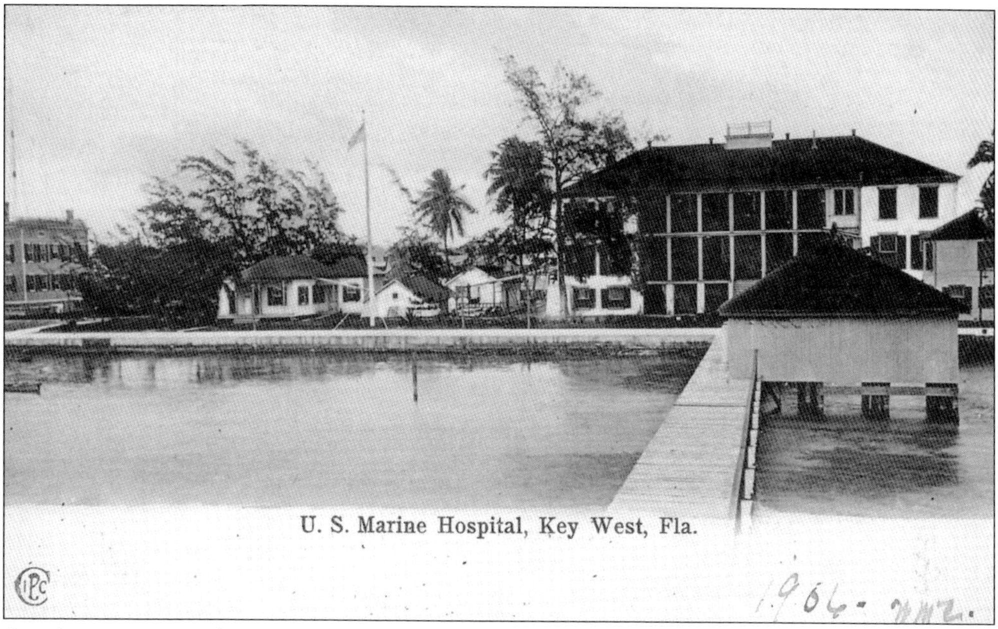
U. S. Marine Hospital, Key West, Fla.

Another common element and a similar design for both the Portsmouth and Key West US Marine Hospitals, seen in this 1906 image, included a pier, making shore access easier and faster. The hospital was seized by Confederate forces but abandoned to Federal forces by early 1862. The hospital resumed service as a US Marine Hospital in 1865. However, the geographical change and depressed postwar economy dramatically slowed shipping in the area, and the hospital closed in 1872.

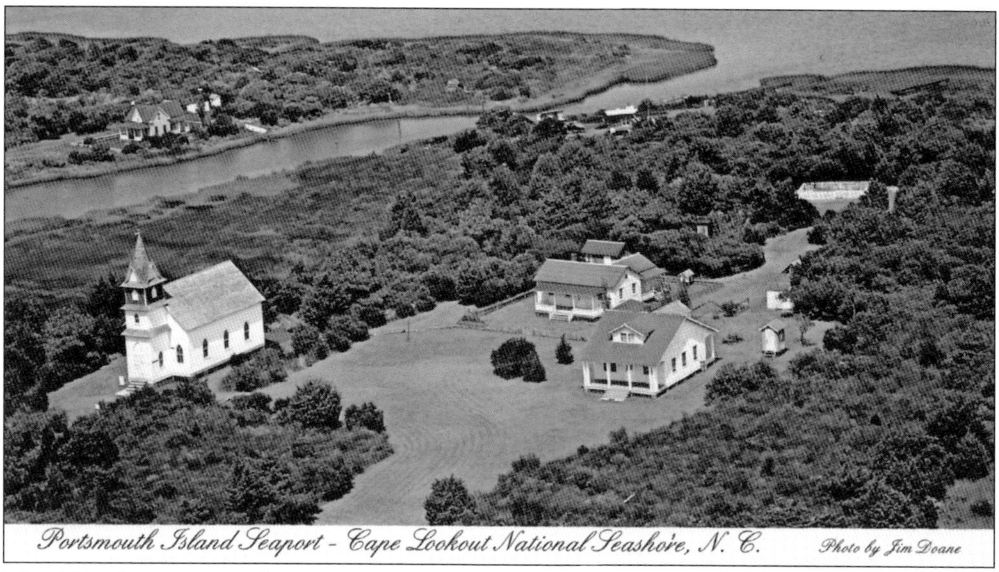
Portsmouth Island Seaport - Cape Lookout National Seashore, N. C.
Photo by Jim Doane

The 1846 hurricane and the war doomed the Ocracoke Port and Portsmouth Village. The hospital sat vacant across from the soon-to-open US Lifesaving Station when it burned in 1894. By 1972, the last Portsmouth Village resident left the island, and it became part of the Cape Lookout National Seashore. Although the hospital property (the cistern is all that remains today) and lifesaving station are just southeast and out of the frame shown here, pictured is most of what remains of the village.

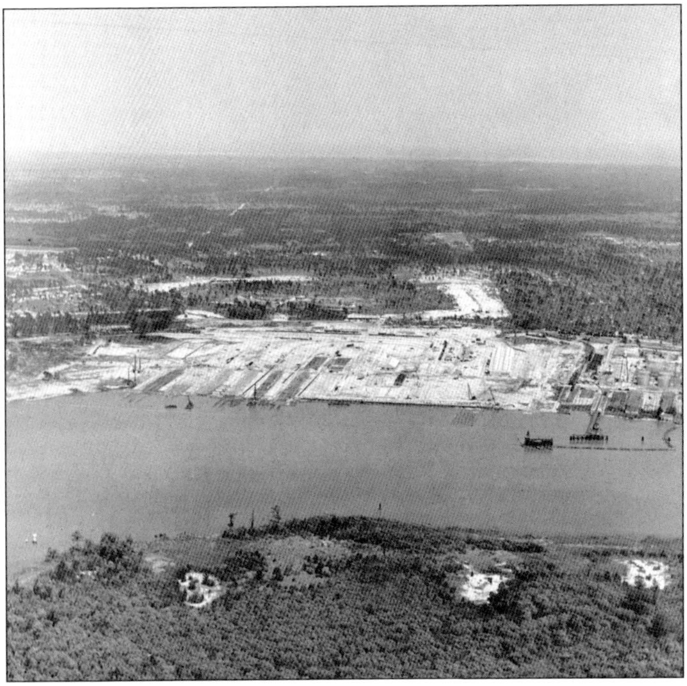

The Wilmington Marine Hospital Association was established in December 1835. The association purchased the Mount Tirzah plantation from recently elected governor Edward Dudley. In 1843, the Seaman's Friend Society organized and built the Seaman's Bethel at Front and Dock Streets. In April 1855, the Wilmington Marine Hospital Association transferred the Mount Tirzah property to the Seaman's Friend Society. By the 1940s, this property (pictured here) became the future state port and a shipbuilding facility.

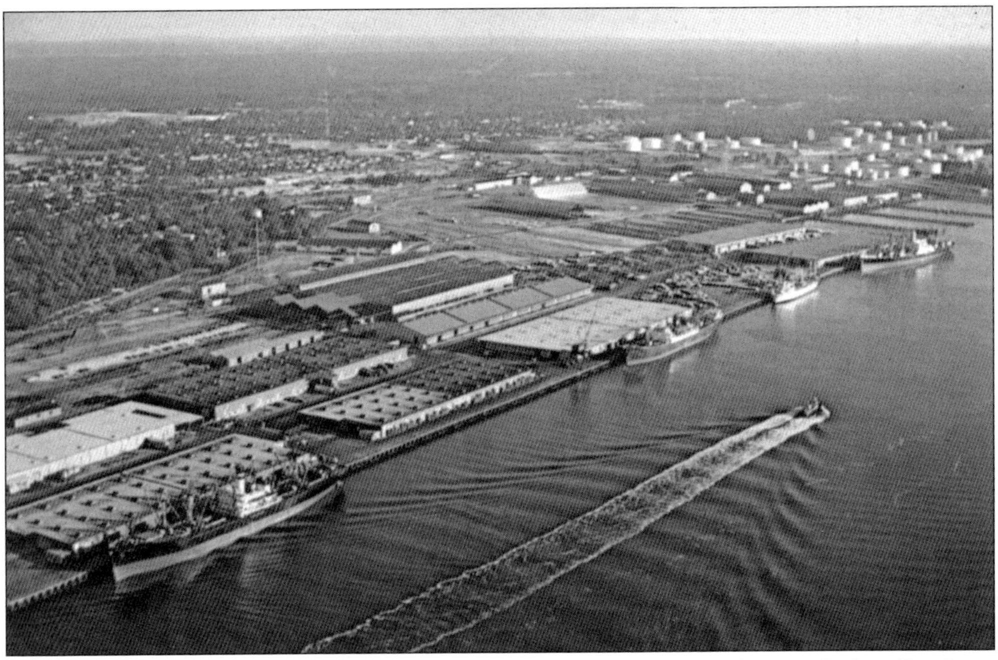

The location identified on a 1860s map as "Hospital Point" is today the North Carolina State Port property. The association converted the property into a quarantine hospital (referred to as a lazaretto) for sick seamen. During the American Civil War, the Mount Tirzah lazaretto burned to the ground. Following the war, another building on the Mount Tirzah property was used for a lazaretto during the 1865 smallpox outbreak. On a 1892 map, it was identified as the "Quarantine Hospital" and was occasionally used by the city government as a pesthouse until it burned in 1898.

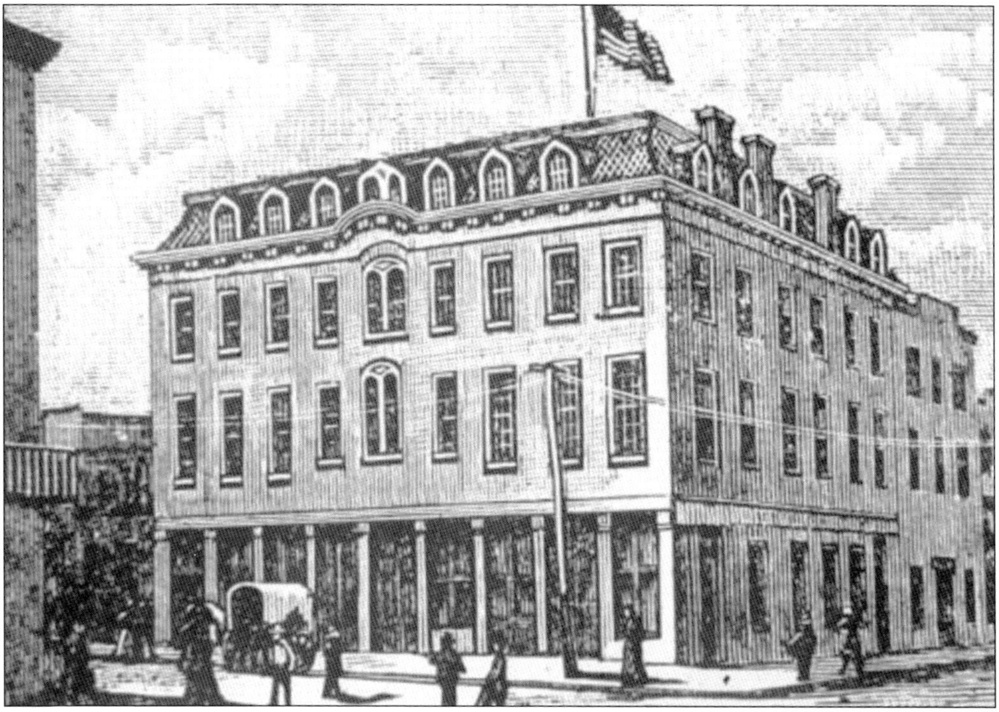

In 1843, the Seaman's Friend Society organized and built the Seaman's Bethel at Front and Dock Streets. During the American Civil War, the Seaman's Bethel was "loaned" to the Confederate government and used as a hospital. It became Confederate General Hospital No. 4 with Dr. H.J. Macon as the commanding surgeon. When the city fell to Federal troops in 1865, for a time, the Seaman's Bethel was used as a Union hospital for black troops before later returning to use as a bethel. (New Hanover County Public Library.)

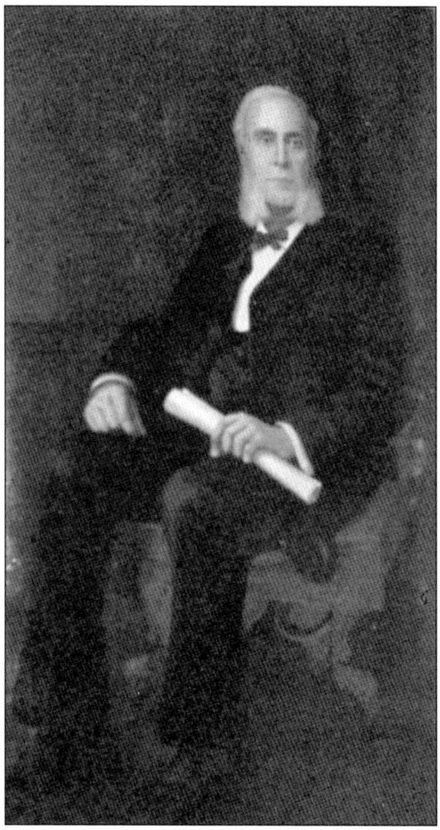

James B. Walker was born in Scotland in 1821. He was living in Richmond, Virginia, and was a successful construction contractor before moving to Wilmington when he was awarded the contract to build a US Marine Hospital. He later built additional hospitals, but his final contribution was the hospital he personally partially funded; it was named for him. Sadly, he died just months before it opened in 1901.

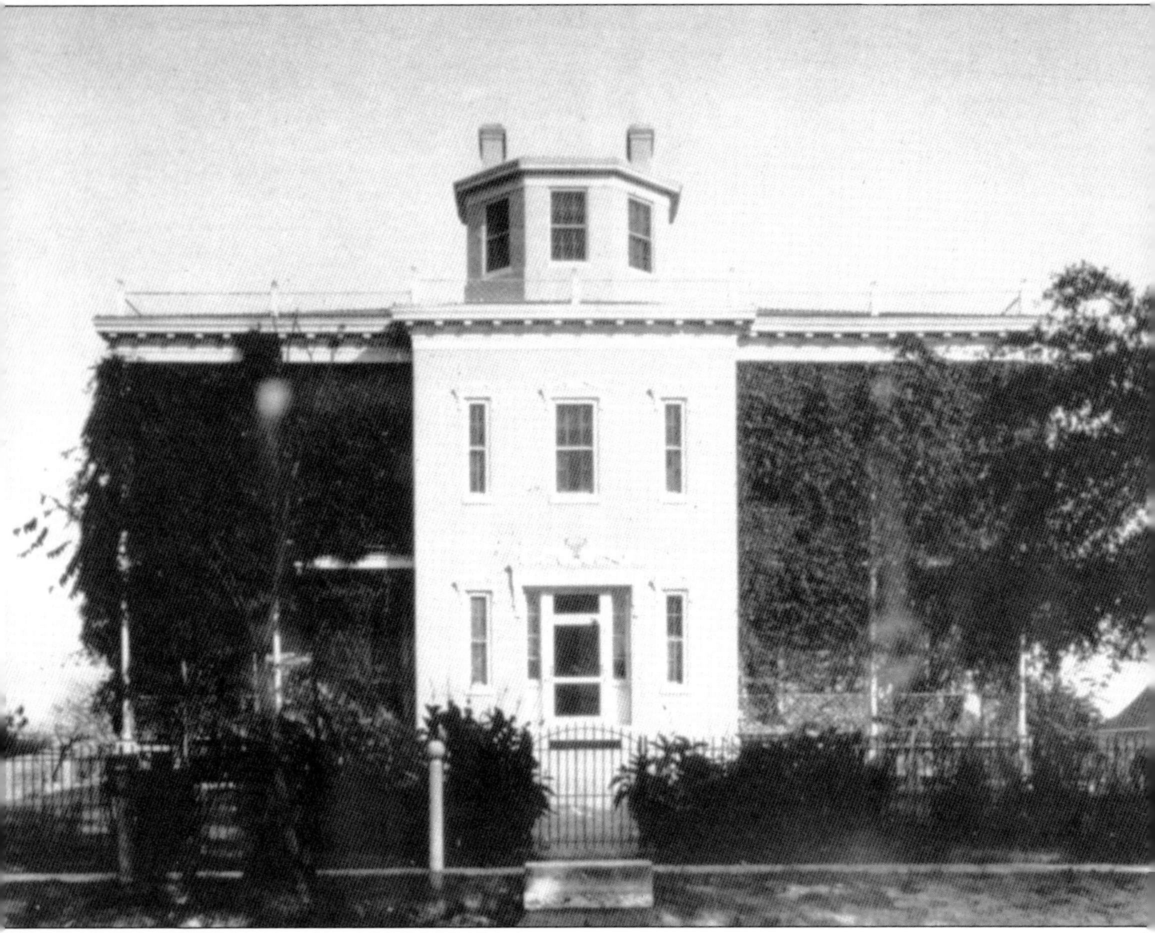

The US Marine Hospital in Wilmington was built in the block bordered by Eighth, Nun, Thirteenth, and Ann Streets. In 1861, the Confederate government seized the hospital, and it became Confederate General Hospital No. 5. The medical records of the 2nd North Carolina Regiment from 1862 to 1864 show 2,180 men used this hospital. The medical officer (surgeon) was Dr. T.R. Micks. In 1865, when the Union army captured Wilmington, this hospital was used for Union troops. While the hospital played multiple roles during the American Civil War and in the years that followed during the occupation, between the depressed economy and the emergence of civilian hospitals, demand for the service continued to decline until it ultimately closed. The hospital building was torn down in 1951. (New Hanover County Public Library.)

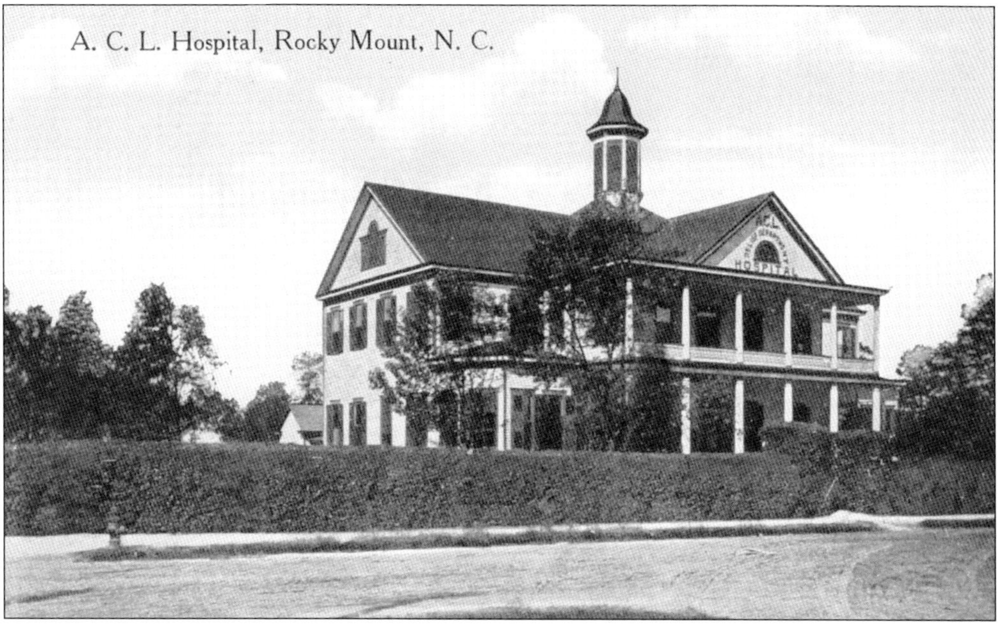

In 1892, the ACL Relief Department Hospital was built in Rocky Mount (which borders Nash and Edgecombe Counties) for employees and their dependents. A major railroad of the time was the Atlantic Coast Line (ACL). The 35-bed hospital opened in 1899 under the direction of Dr. E.B. Quillen in 1906. The hospital was lost to fire later in the 1920s.

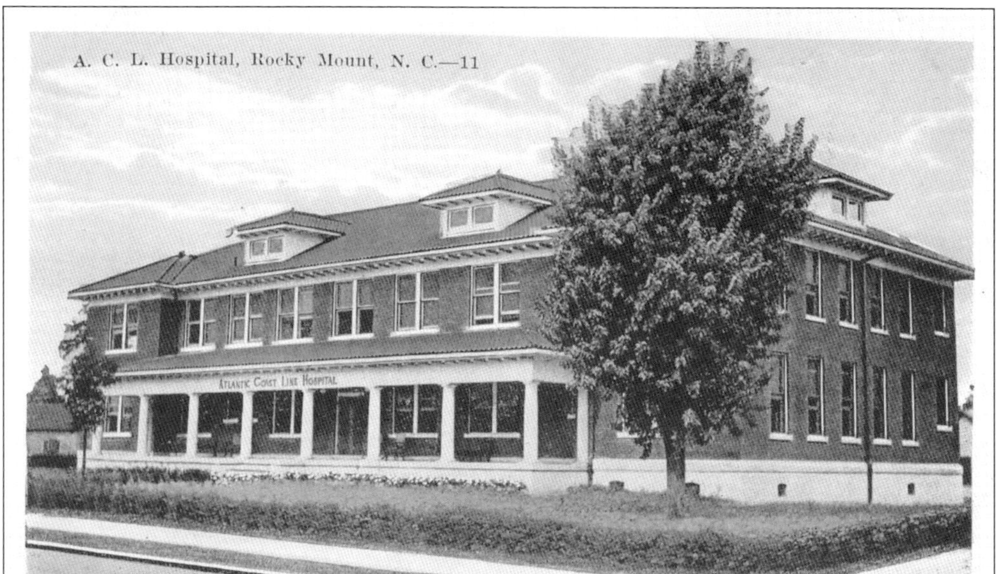

This building replaced the original ACL Relief Department Hospital. This was one of two ACL hospitals (with the other being at Waycross, Georgia). Headquartered in Wilmington, the ACL had a major interchange with other rail lines in Rocky Mount leading to Richmond and Portsmouth, Virginia. The hospital closed around 1963 when the ACL began to use local health care facilities for their employees and dependents.

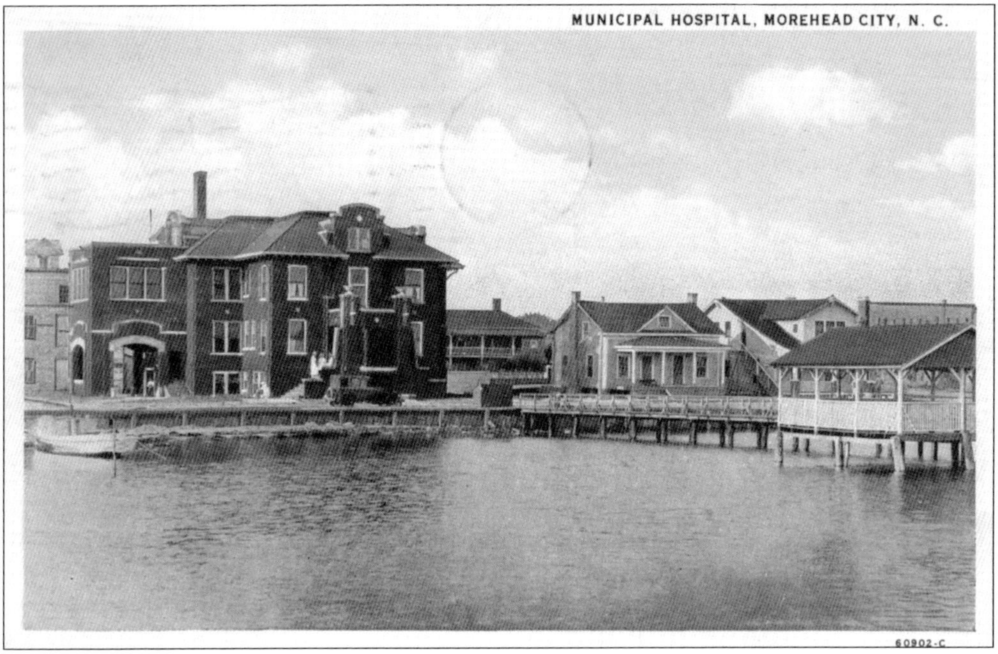

The Municipal Hospital of Morehead City in Carteret County was established in 1911, near the port. The hospital was built with a pier for ships coming to port with sick and injured seamen to be ferried there as well as others who primarily traveled the area by boat.

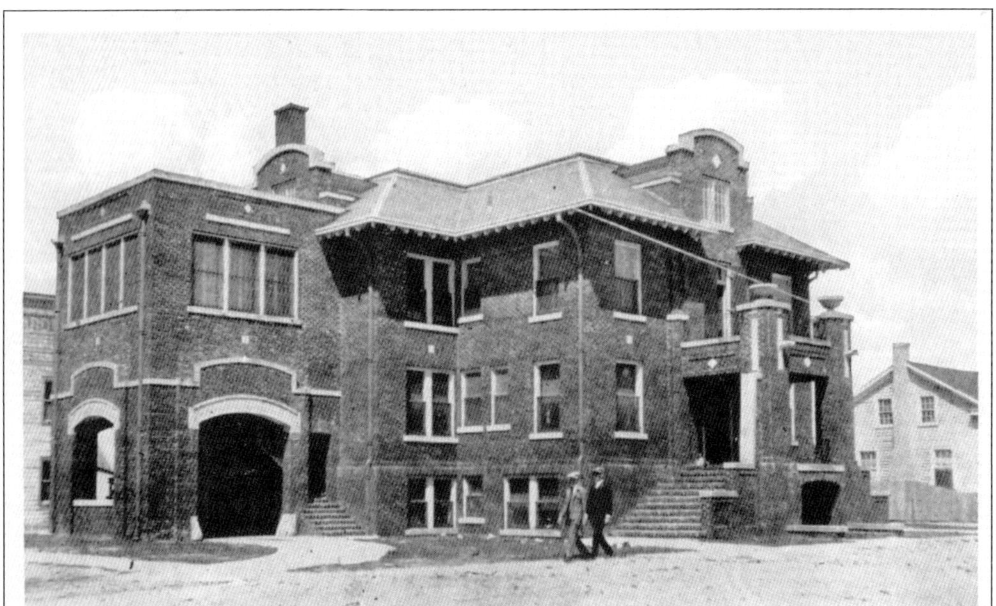

Here is another view of the Municipal Hospital of Morehead City, which included a covered area to unload and load patients. By 1923, this 35-bed hospital was led by Dr. Ben Royal (surgeon).

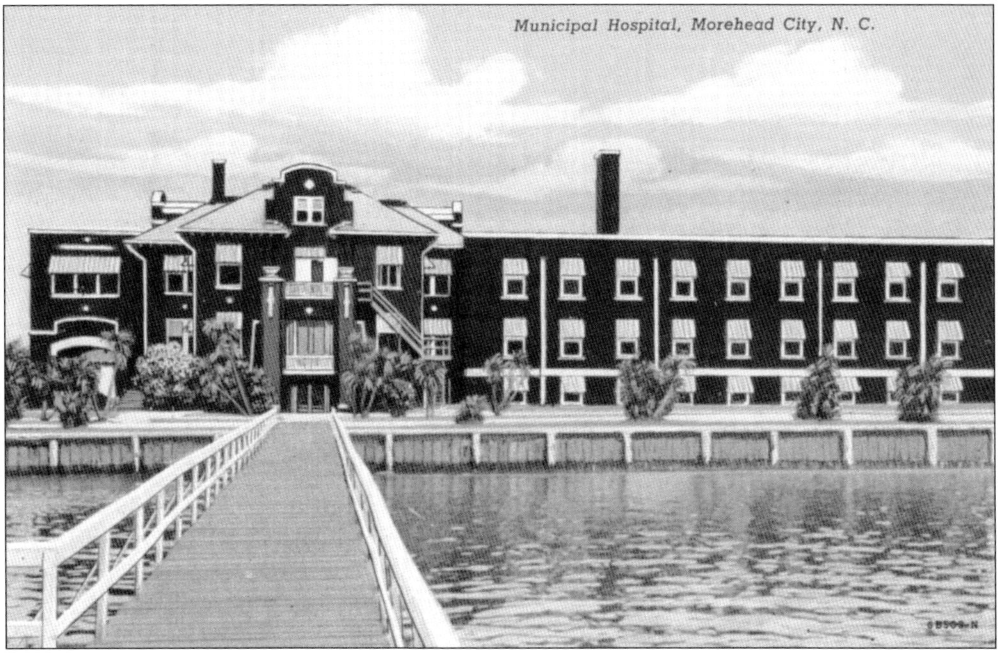

Seen above is a view of the Municipal Hospital featuring a long pier and the original hospital structure along with a wing added in the early 1950s (section to the right of the main building). The hospital was later replaced with the creation of Carteret General Hospital, which opened in 1967. (Today, it is known as Carteret Health Care System.)

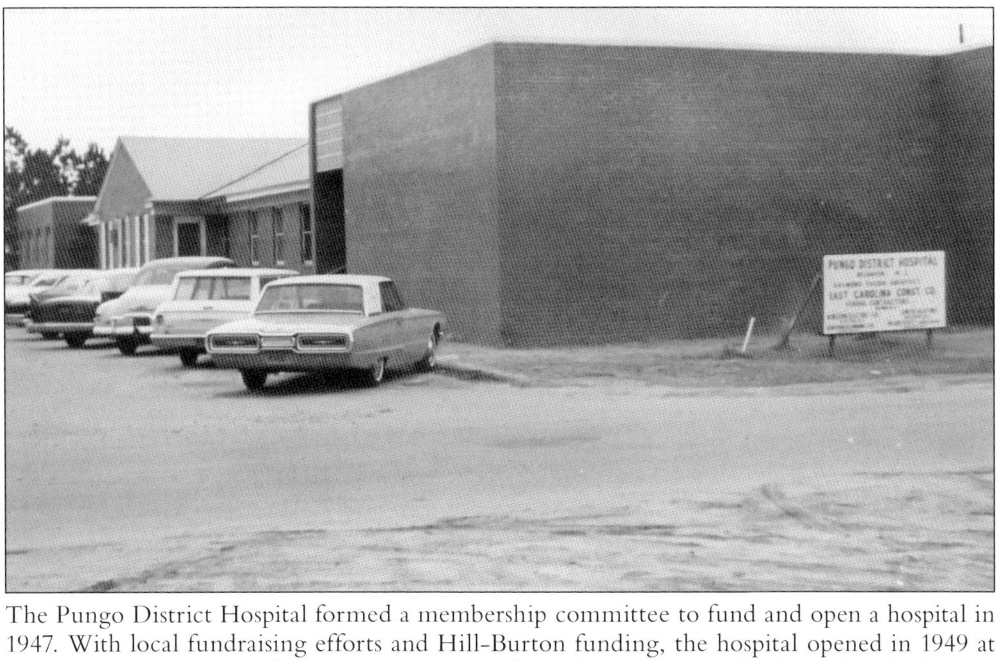

The Pungo District Hospital formed a membership committee to fund and open a hospital in 1947. With local fundraising efforts and Hill-Burton funding, the hospital opened in 1949 at 202 East Water Street, Belhaven. It served part of Beaufort County and mainland Hyde County residents. The 49-bed hospital gained CAH designation but still financially struggled. After a 2011 merger with Vidant Health amid ongoing losses, Vidant closed the hospital. (North Carolina State Archives.)

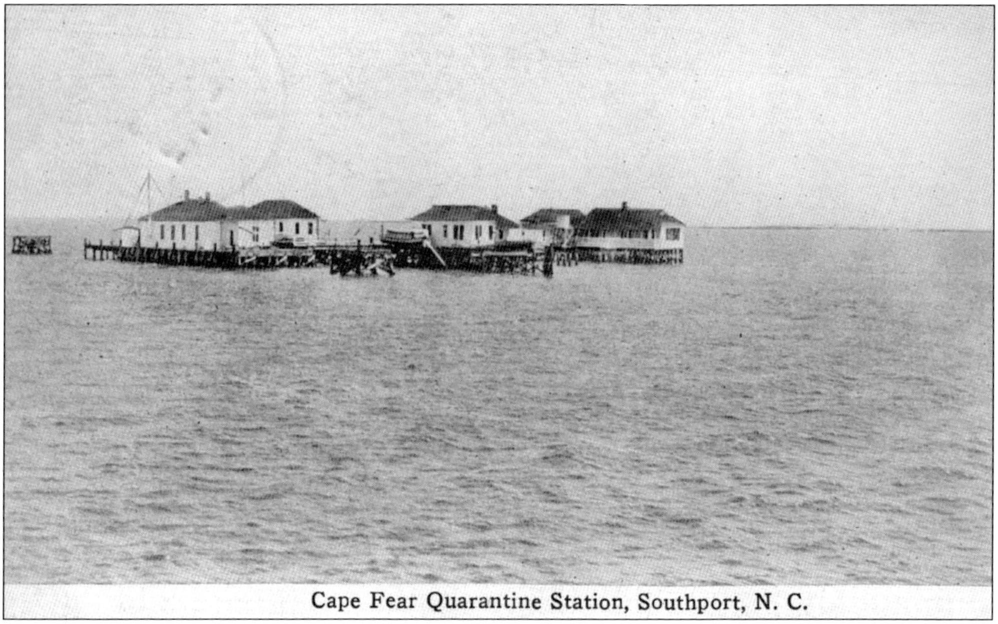

In 1882, the original Smithville quarantine station was destroyed by fire (Smithville was renamed Southport in 1887). Although beset by several delays, the US Marine Hospital Service authorized construction of a replacement facility. Completed in 1897, it was located just offshore (upriver near Price's Creek Lighthouse). This c. 1907 image included buildings described as quarters for detained sailors, a hospital, and a wharf.

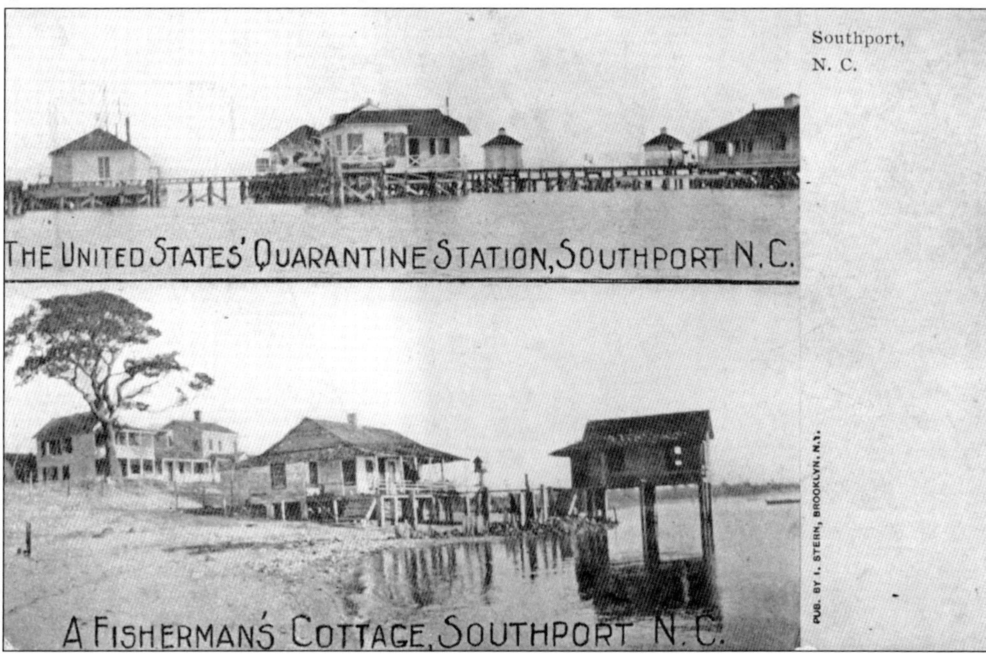

Another view of the Southport US Quarantine Station is shown above. The station was led by Dr. Julius Arthur Dosher, who served as the acting assistant surgeon in the US Public Health Service. By the mid-1930s, the quarantine process was replaced by international public health laws for international trade. The station closed in 1937.

Four

"Colored" Sanatoriums and Hospitals

While the American Civil War settled one great injustice, another began to arise in the decades that followed. State-sponsored racial segregation was codified by law following the 1896 landmark US Supreme Court decision *Plessy v. Ferguson* (establishing the legal basis for separate but equal). The outcome in Eastern North Carolina was similar to many other communities throughout the United States and particularly the traditional Southern states. Racial segregation spawned the creation of "colored" or "negro" asylums, sanatoriums, clinics, and hospitals. Even in health care, separate was seldom equal.

Segregated health care was the norm for the first half of the 20th century. This included hospitals and doctors' offices and extended into waiting rooms, water fountains, restrooms, and patient wards. In several communities, the solution was to create a "blacks-only" hospital or clinic.

The antidiscrimination aspect of Medicare and Medicaid was the ultimate driving force behind consolidating smaller, often race-specific hospitals and ending the racial divide at hospitals. Where services were under the same roof, segregation may have been a subtle divide such as separate entrances to the hospital and separate restrooms and cafeteria accommodations. It may have been more overt such as denying hospital privileges to physicians who were "colored." Regardless, Medicare was a strong driver of change regarding how health care was going to be funded and required the end to all matters related to divisions based on race.

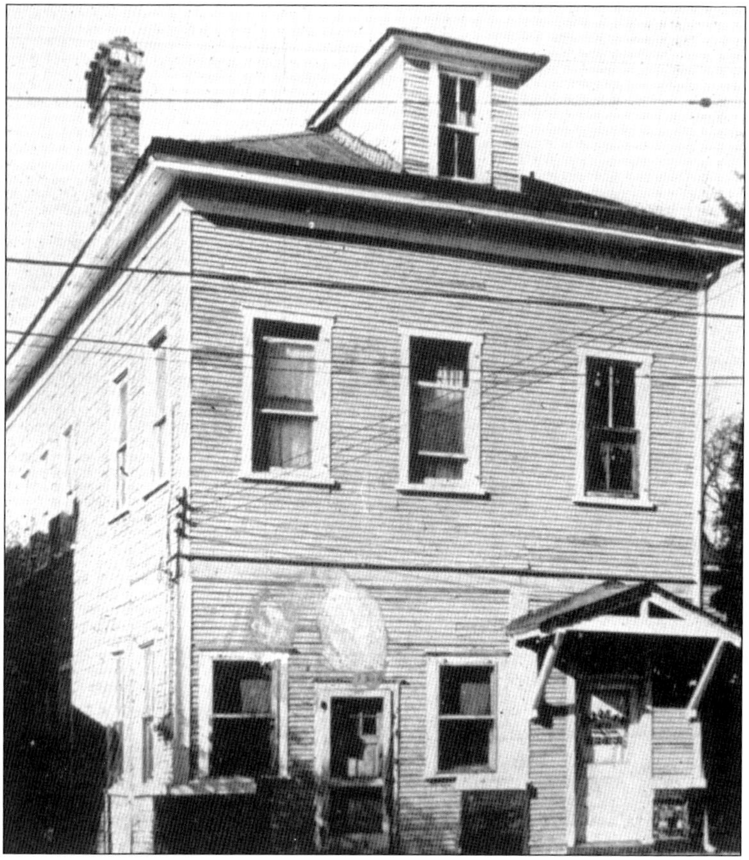

The Community Hospital opened in 1920 at 415 North Seventh Street. While the two Wilmington hospitals offered "colored beds" or "colored wards," only white physicians had privileges to see patients in those hospitals. Seven African American physicians organized a medical society, raised funds, and purchased the Niestlie Drug Store. It became their first hospital building. By 1923, this was a 50-bed hospital, led by Dr. Foster F. Burnett, who was the PIC. (New Hanover County Public Library.)

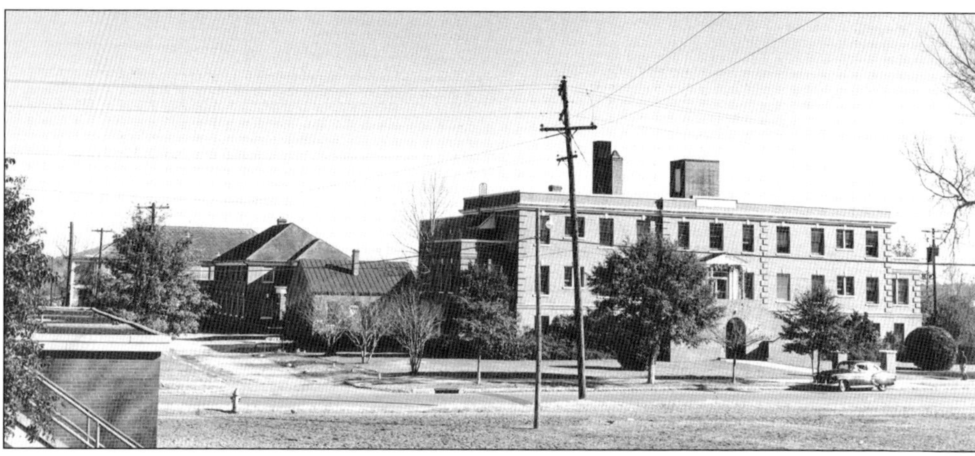

The new Community Hospital building opened in 1939 on South Eleventh Street. A nursing education program also began at the hospital. Community Hospital served "colored patients" of the Greater Wilmington area until a community bond was passed to build a large regional hospital in 1961. It closed in 1966, along with the James Walker Memorial Hospital, and patients were moved to the New Hanover Memorial Hospital. (New Hanover County Public Library.)

In 1912, the Wilson Hospital and Tubercular Home/Mercy Hospital opened on East Green Street. This was the first hospital for "colored only" in the region. By 1923, it had 16 beds and 12 TB beds, and Dr. F.S. Hargrave was the PIC. The hospital closed in 1964 when the area hospitals merged into one large general hospital, Wilson Memorial. (Digital NC, Wilson County Public Library.)

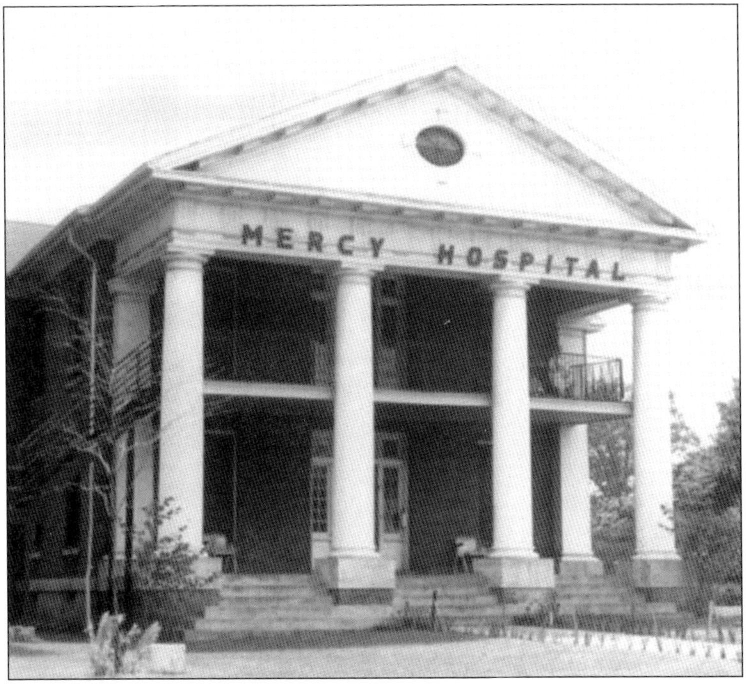

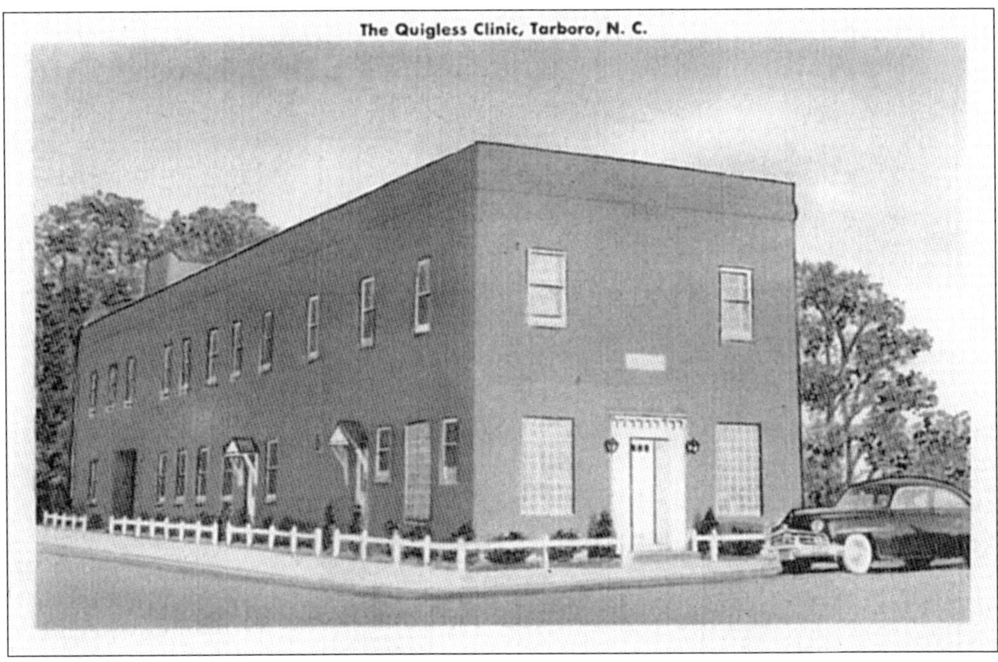

Dr. Milton Quigless opened the Quigless Clinic (hospital) in 1946 in Tarboro (Edgecombe County) to serve everyone. Described on the card as a 26-bed hospital for "Negros," it operated from 1946 to 1974 until the services were consolidated with the local general hospital. It was located at the corner of Main and St. Andrews Streets (99 Main Street in Tarboro), at the roundabout adjacent to the Tar River Bridge across from Princeville. Today, the building is a multiuse office. (Image 39177 from the East Carolina University Digital Collections.)

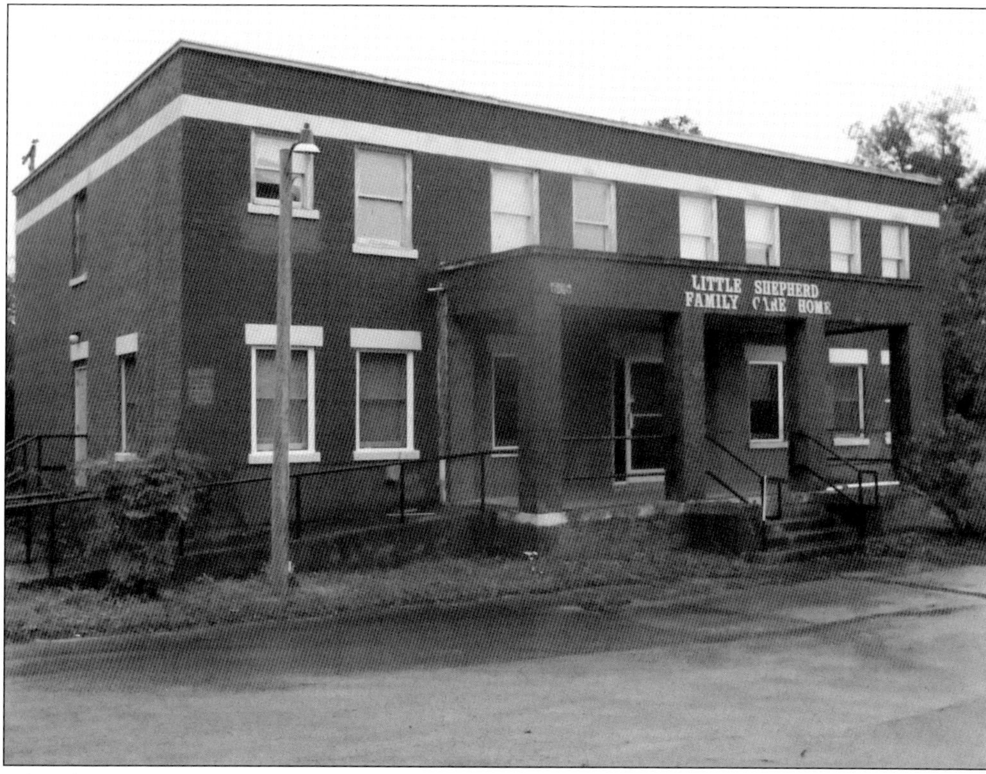

After the 1922 New Bern fire, Reverend Johnson of St. Cyprian Church realized the need for a hospital for "black people." In 1938, the Episcopal Diocese built the Good Shepherd Hospital at 603 West Street (and provided ongoing support). By 1956, it was a 58-bed general hospital with eight bassinets. The hospital closed in 1962 when the patients were transferred to the new Craven Memorial Hospital.

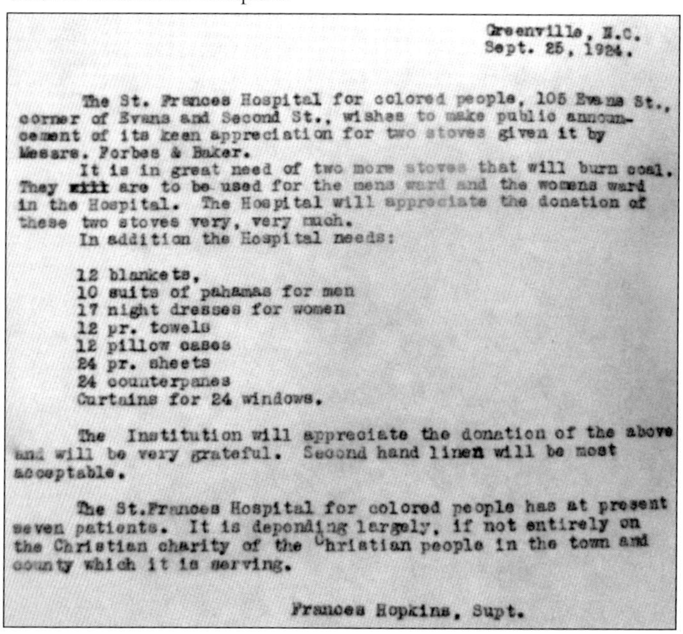

Greenville, N.C.
Sept. 25, 1924.

The St. Frances Hospital for colored people, 105 Evans St., corner of Evans and Second St., wishes to make public announcement of its keen appreciation for two stoves given it by Messrs. Forbes & Baker.

It is in great need of two more stoves that will burn coal. They ~~will~~ are to be used for the mens ward and the womens ward in the Hospital. The Hospital will appreciate the donation of these two stoves very, very much.

In addition the Hospital needs:

12 blankets,
10 suits of pahamas for men
17 night dresses for women
12 pr. towels
12 pillow cases
24 pr. sheets
24 counterpanes
Curtains for 24 windows.

The Institution will appreciate the donation of the above and will be very grateful. Second hand linen will be most acceptable.

The St.Frances Hospital for colored people has at present seven patients. It is depending largely, if not entirely on the Christian charity of the Christian people in the town and county which it is serving.

Frances Hopkins, Supt.

St. Francis Hospital opened at 105 Evans Street (at the corner of Second Street) for "colored people" in Greenville. In September 1924, the Greenville Kiwanis began fundraising for a "colored hospital." Frances Hopkins, a black nurse, had operated a two-bed hospital in her home at 114 North Washington Street. Patients needing surgery were transported to Community Hospital by ambulance and returned following the surgery. (Sheppard Memorial Library/*A Tradition of Excellence PCMH*.)

Five

American Civil War Hospitals

By early 1862, with North Carolina's accessibility by train from the Virginia and Maryland battlefields, the area became a prime location for Confederate hospitals. Trains were used to shuttle the sick and injured from the temporary battlefield hospitals to more permanent ones. As the war began, volunteers were organized in several cities, including Raleigh and Wilmington. By the end of the war, tens of thousands had volunteered to care for the sick and wounded, and local buildings such as hotels, churches, and schools were converted to hospitals, surrounded by tents for the overflow of patients.

While certainly not all-inclusive, this chapter includes examples of the five types of hospitals used. The "general hospitals" were for those with more serious injuries or illnesses. Most of these were buildings previously used as colleges or private schools that were turned over to the Confederate government and converted to hospitals. Additional buildings located along major rail lines were adopted as "wayside hospitals," meaning that a soldier could rest or recover there. The coastal forts included a designated "fort hospital" area. As the battlefields moved, "field hospitals" were quickly created close to where the fighting was taking place to care for the wounded. It was hoped that the selected location was far enough behind the lines for safety. With these rapidly changing conditions and this massive surge of injuries following frequent engagements, both armies routinely seized churches, schools, private homes, and government buildings for "temporary hospitals."

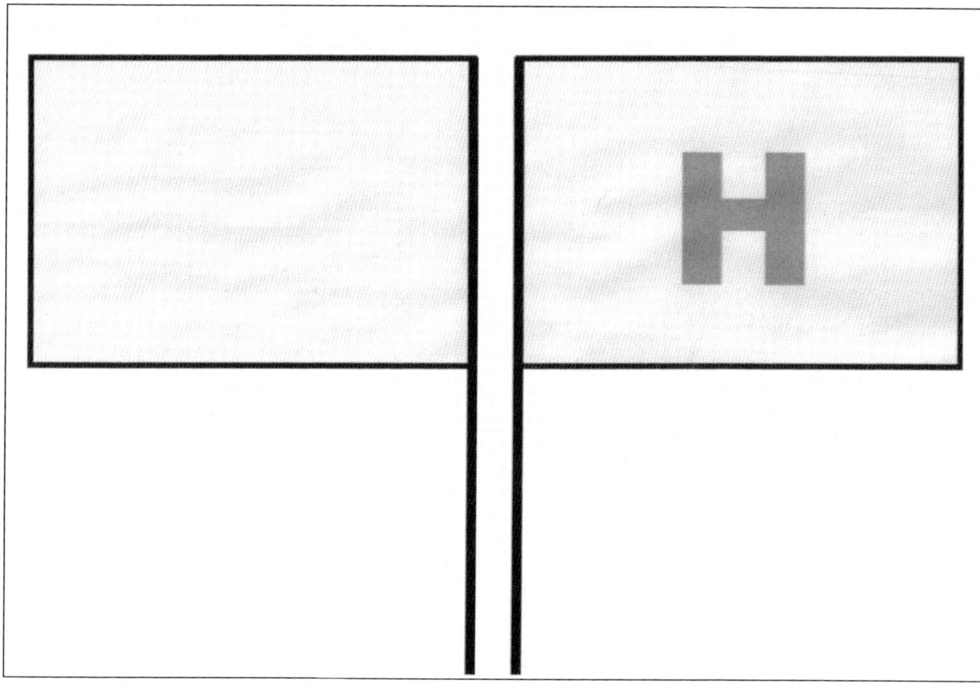

Confederate and Union hospitals were marked by a large yellow flag. By 1864, the Union had added a large green "H" to the center of their hospital flags. Confederate hospitals were managed by a surgeon, who was assisted by aides or nurses, who were either military personnel or area volunteers. Union hospitals were similarly managed by a surgeon and nurse volunteers either from the area or brought there from Northern churches.

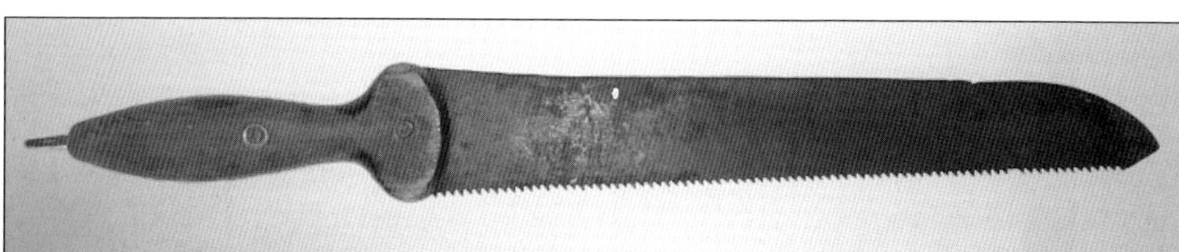

A by-product of war is many patients in short periods of time. This promotes rapid development of tools and procedures used to improve outcomes and reduce mortality. By the end of the American Civil War, amputations could be completed in minutes with minimal complications. This commonly used bone saw includes a smooth side for cutting tissue and a sawtooth side for more dense material such as bone.

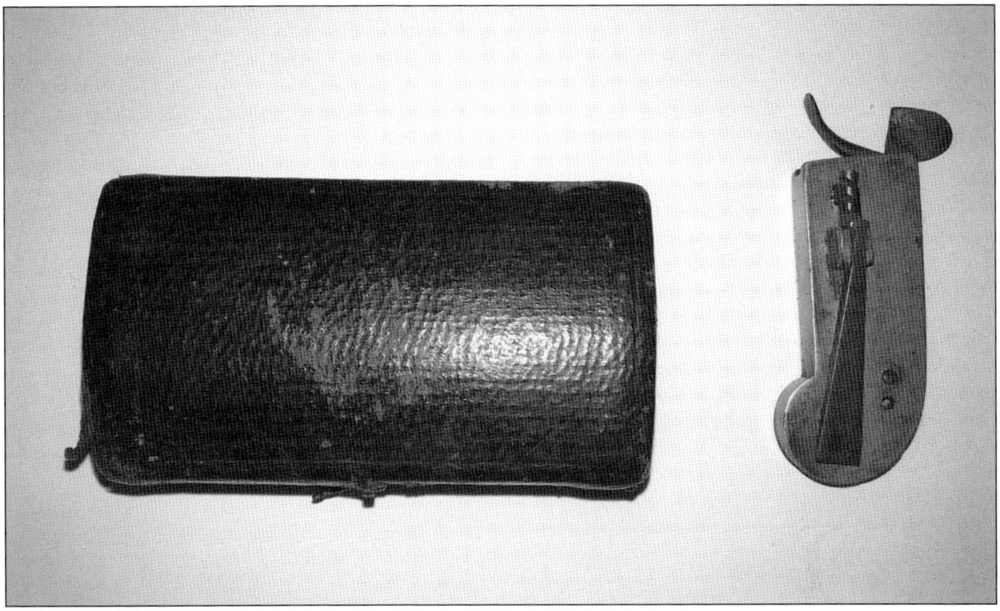

Bloodletting was a common method of treating patients with multiple conditions in the 18th and 19th centuries. This device was a spring-loaded cutter designed to minimize the pain associated with cutting the patient. Bloodletting was once a treatment for most any condition—infection, trauma, childbirth, headache, cancer, etc.

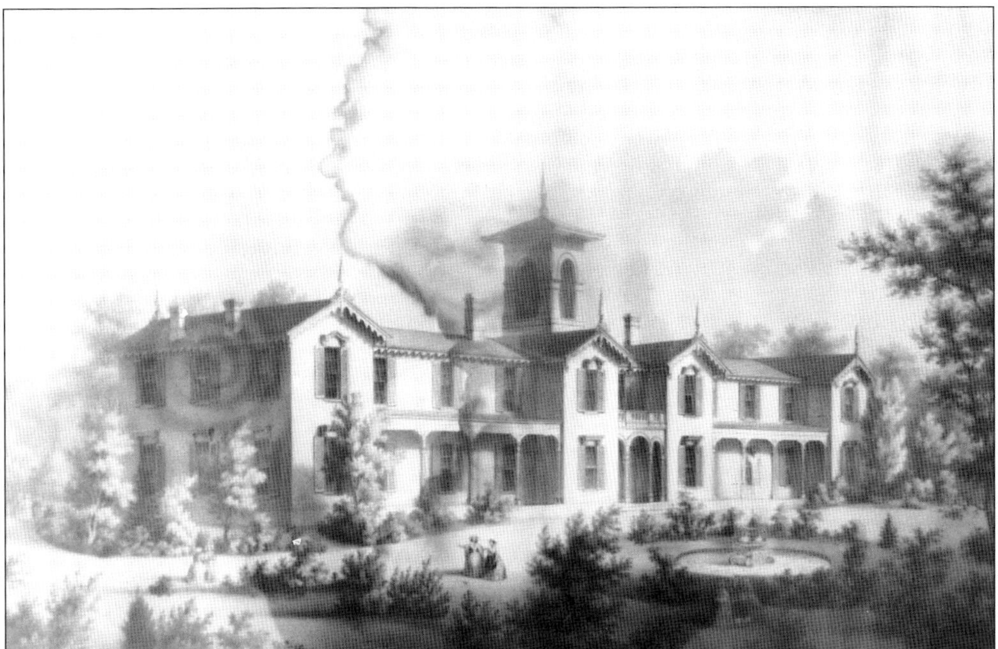

In April 1862, the Confederate government converted the Wilson Female Academy, at Herring Avenue and Gold Street, next to the Wilmington-Weldon Railroad, into Confederate General Hospital No. 2. This location was ideal to manage soldiers from Virginia battlefields. The hospital was led by chief surgeon Dr. Solomon Sampson Satchwell. After the war, the building became the Wilson Collegiate Institute from 1872 until 1898. (Wilson County Public Library.)

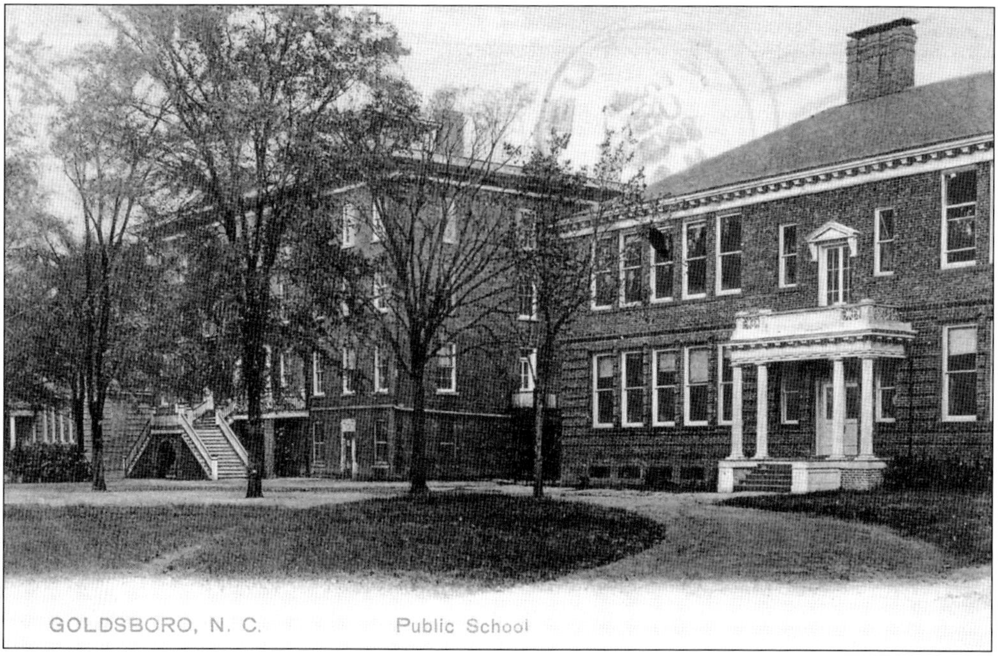

In 1861, the Confederate government converted the Goldsborough Female Academy (center building) on North Williams Street into Confederate General Hospital No. 3, led by chief surgeon W.A. Holt. The Wilmington port and the Eastern North Carolina railroads connected at Goldsborough, making the city an ideal location for a large hospital. In March 1865, Sherman's Union army targeted the city, the last major supply line to Lee's Army of Northern Virginia.

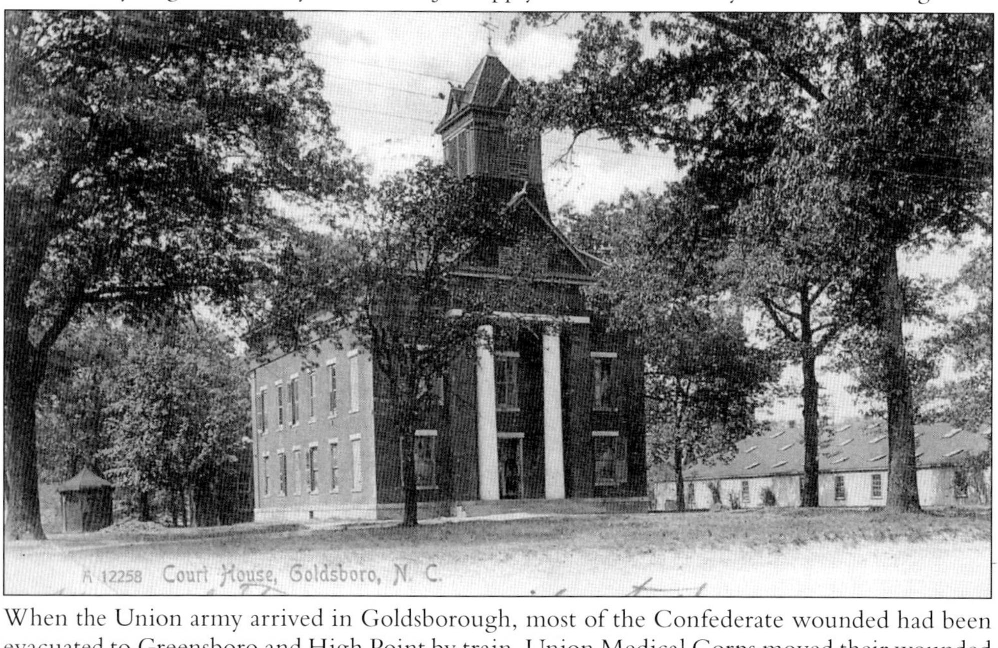

When the Union army arrived in Goldsborough, most of the Confederate wounded had been evacuated to Greensboro and High Point by train. Union Medical Corps moved their wounded into Confederate General Hospital No. 2 for continued care as General Sherman, for a time, occupied the city. The Union wounded from Bentonville overfilled the hospital, and the local courthouse was also commandeered by the Union Medical Corps.

The Roanoke River divides the towns of Weldon (Halifax County) and Garysburg (Northampton County). At the onset of the war, multiple railroads connected here, including Wilmington-Weldon, Seaboard & Roanoke, Petersburg, and Raleigh & Gaston Railroads. The Garysburg Methodist Church was used as a wayside hospital. The medical officer was surgeon H.H. Hunter. A military cemetery was created in Weldon, at West First and Rosemary Streets.

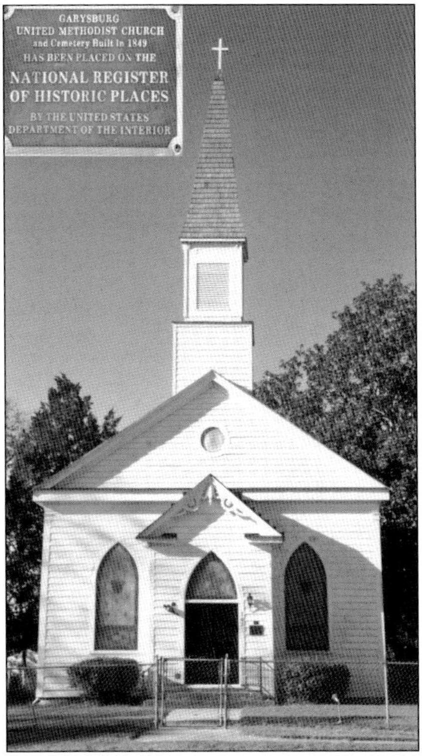

GARYSBURG
UNITED METHODIST CHURCH
and Cemetery Built In 1849
HAS BEEN PLACED ON THE
NATIONAL REGISTER
OF HISTORIC PLACES
BY THE UNITED STATES
DEPARTMENT OF THE INTERIOR

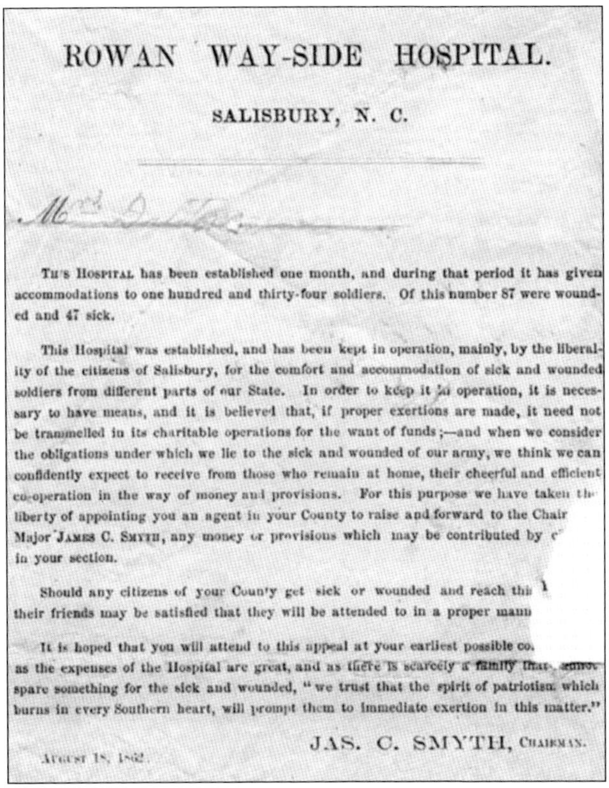

ROWAN WAY-SIDE HOSPITAL.

SALISBURY, N. C.

Mrs D. ...

This Hospital has been established one month, and during that period it has given accommodations to one hundred and thirty-four soldiers. Of this number 87 were wounded and 47 sick.

This Hospital was established, and has been kept in operation, mainly, by the liberality of the citizens of Salisbury, for the comfort and accommodation of sick and wounded soldiers from different parts of our State. In order to keep it in operation, it is necessary to have means, and it is believed that, if proper exertions are made, it need not be trammelled in its charitable operations for the want of funds;—and when we consider the obligations under which we lie to the sick and wounded of our army, we think we can confidently expect to receive from those who remain at home, their cheerful and efficient co-operation in the way of money and provisions. For this purpose we have taken the liberty of appointing you an agent in your County to raise and forward to the Chair Major James C. Smyth, any money or provisions which may be contributed by c[illegible] in your section.

Should any citizens of your County get sick or wounded and reach thi[illegible] their friends may be satisfied that they will be attended to in a proper mann[illegible]

It is hoped that you will attend to this appeal at your earliest possible co[illegible] as the expenses of the Hospital are great, and as there is scarcely a family that [illegible] spare something for the sick and wounded, "we trust that the spirit of patriotism which burns in every Southern heart, will prompt them to immediate exertion in this matter."

JAS. C. SMYTH, Chairman.

August 18, 1862.

The wayside hospital served as a treatment center for soldiers with less serious injuries or those who could not be managed in the general hospitals because of overcrowding. It was also a rest and recovery point for soldiers heading home for a brief leave. (Wilson Library, UNC-Chapel Hill.)

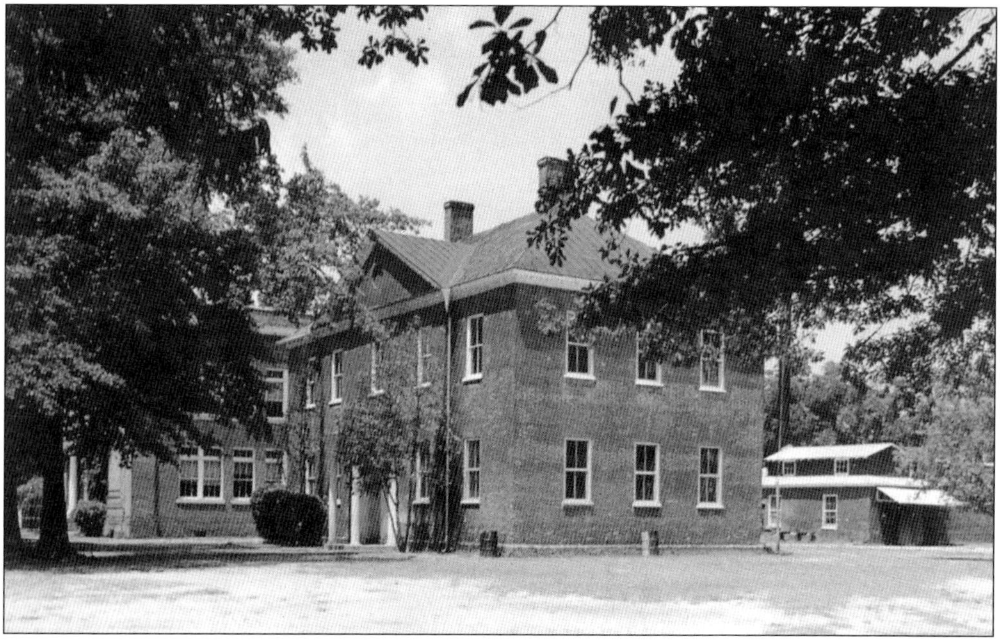

In 1861, the Confederate government converted the New Bern Academy, at 508 New Street, to a hospital. On September 3, 1861, the women of New Bern organized a Soldiers Relief Society to care for sick and wounded troops. Following the Battle of New Bern on March 14, 1862, Union forces captured the city, and the hospital was commandeered to care for the wounded Union troops. Today, the building is a local museum.

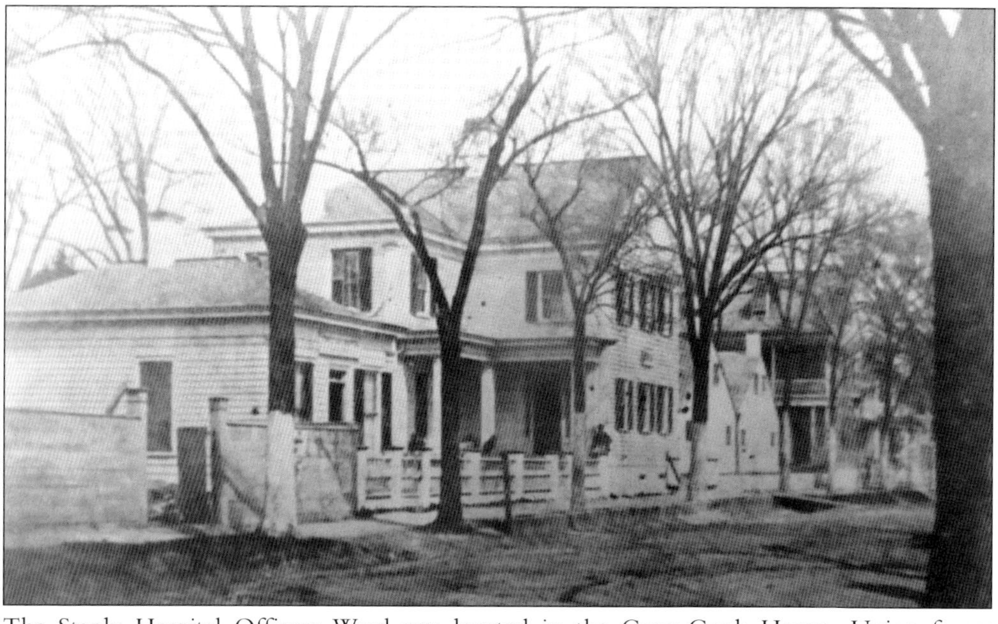

The Stanly Hospital Officers Ward was located in the Coor-Cook House. Union forces occupying New Bern were known as Foster's Volunteers. A multitude of buildings were commandeered for medical services as the number of hospital patients with war wounds and illness grew. The 1865 hospital census reports identified a single hospital of 475 beds as Foster's General Hospital. (UNC North Carolina Collection.)

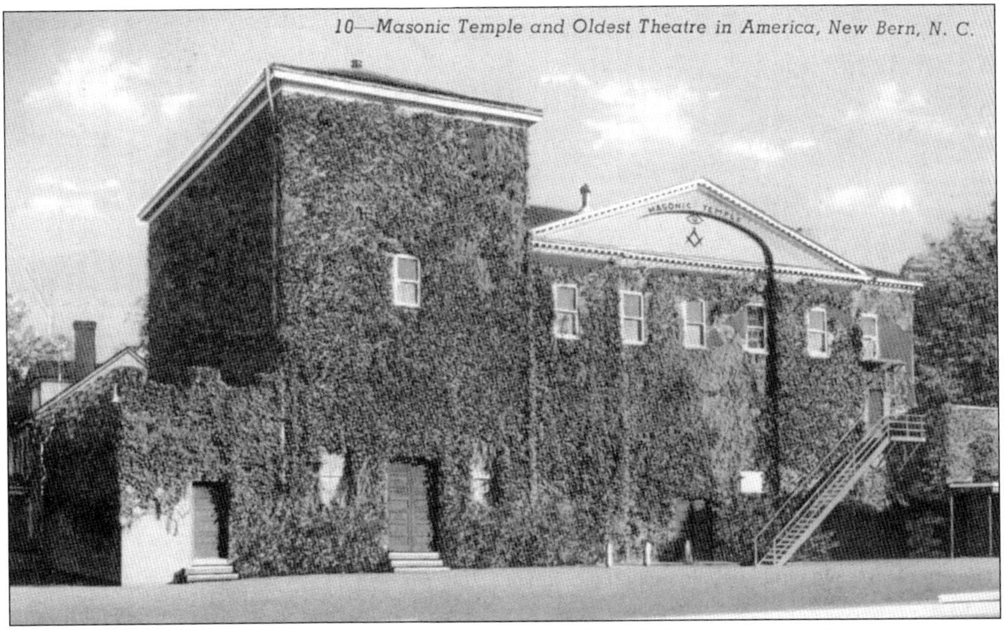
10—Masonic Temple and Oldest Theatre in America, New Bern, N. C.
MASONIC TEMPLE

In early 1865, the New Bern Union Hospital report included one for the Masonic Hospital. By April 1865, more than 2,000 Union soldiers were noted in a consolidated Foster's General Hospital with all the buildings in use at the time. The main building (right side) pictured here includes an addition added after the war (left side).

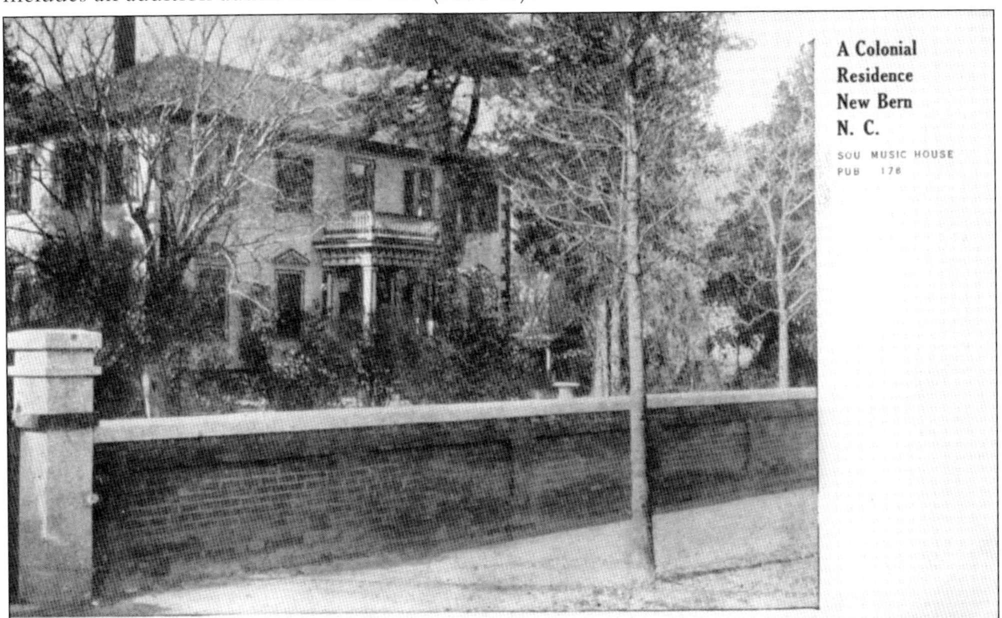
A Colonial
Residence
New Bern
N. C.
SOU MUSIC HOUSE
PUB 176

John Wright Stanly (sometimes Stanley) built this house in 1789. Stanly's ships provided vital supplies to support the American Revolution. When New Bern fell to Union forces on March 1862, Gen. Ambrose Burnside commandeered the house as his headquarters. By October, between war injuries and illness, the house was converted into a third hospital. General Foster authorized the Catholic Sisters to move the Beaufort hospital staff/equipment from Beaufort to this location.

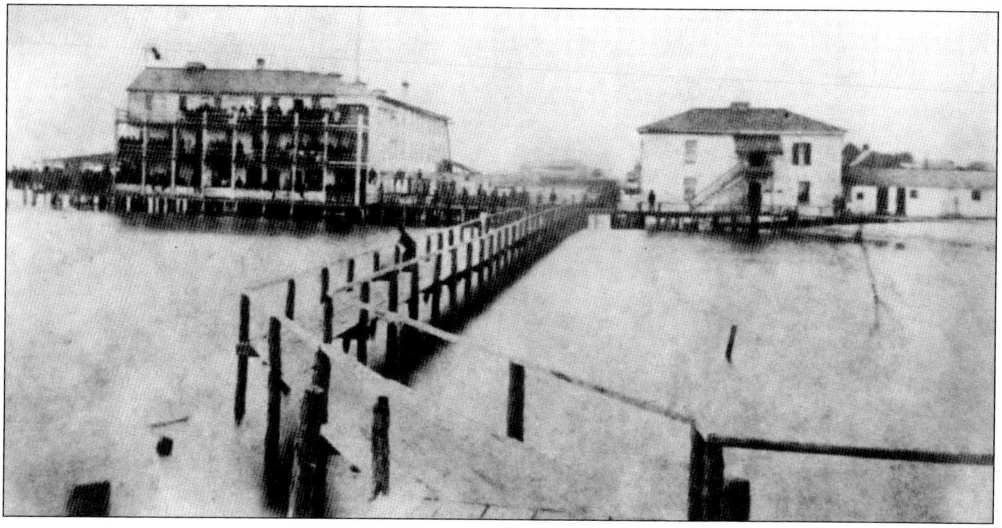

In 1851, the Atlantic House Hotel opened on the Beaufort waterfront (Carteret County). According to a diary kept by the Carteret County clerk of court, James Rumley, the property was seized by Union forces on March 25, 1862. With ongoing battles across the harbor at Fort Macon and just up the river at New Bern, the building was converted by the Union army into the Hammond Hospital. (North Carolina State Archives.)

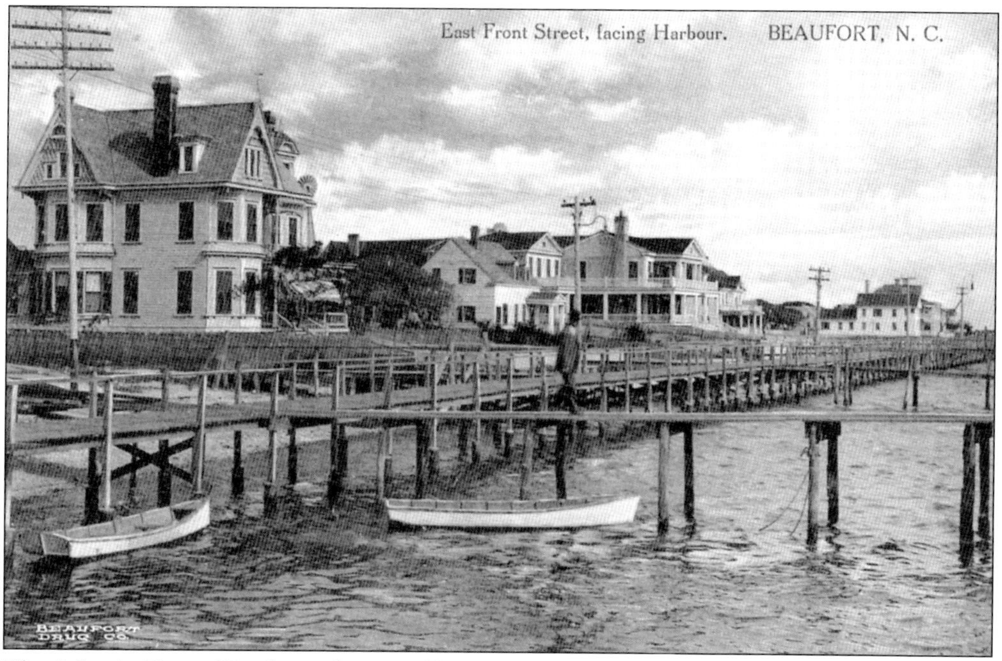
East Front Street, facing Harbour. BEAUFORT, N. C.
BEAUFORT DRUG CO.

The Atlantic House Hotel was destroyed by a storm in 1879. Pictured here around 1905 is the Beaufort waterfront. The large open area on the waterfront in the center of the picture is where the former hospital once stood. On the map, the hotel sat between Pollock and Marsh Streets and just east of the Inlet Inn (also known as Norcom House) on Front Street, generally where a bank is located today.

In 1781, the Wilmington St. James Episcopal Church was used by Lord Cornwallis and the British Army (following the Battle of Moore's Creek) as a military hospital. The 1781 structure was replaced in 1839, at the same location. In 1865, Fort Fisher fell to Union forces protecting the Cape Fear and Wilmington port. Wilmington surrendered seven days later. Union forces used the church as a hospital for their wounded soldiers.

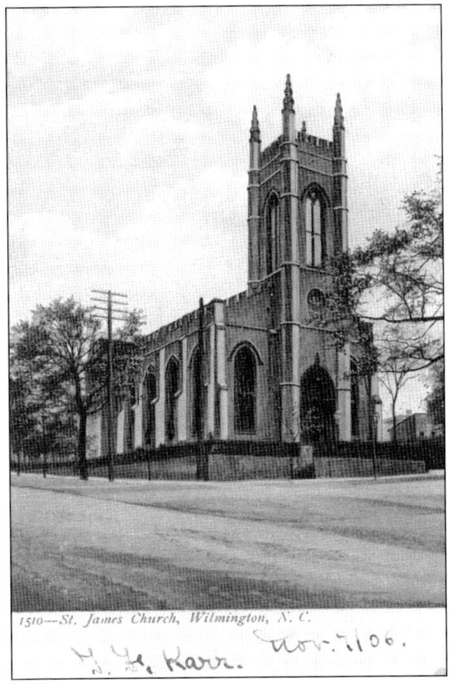

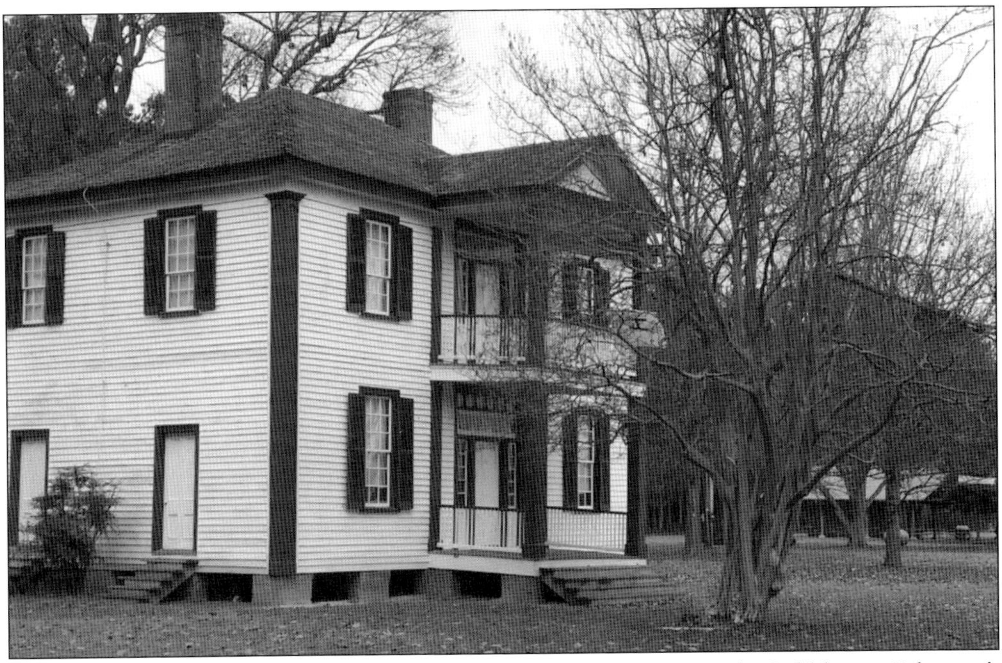

As Sherman's Union forces (more than 50,000) moved toward Goldsboro, Johnston's Confederate forces (approximately 30,000) set up to engage them near Bentonville (Johnston County). As the two great armies began to establish their positions for battle, the Harper House was commandeered by the Federal XIV Corps as a battlefield hospital. Once the battle ended, Union medical personnel transported their wounded following the troop movement to Goldsboro. Forty-five wounded Confederate soldiers remained at the Harper House, cared for by the Harper family and Confederate medical personnel.

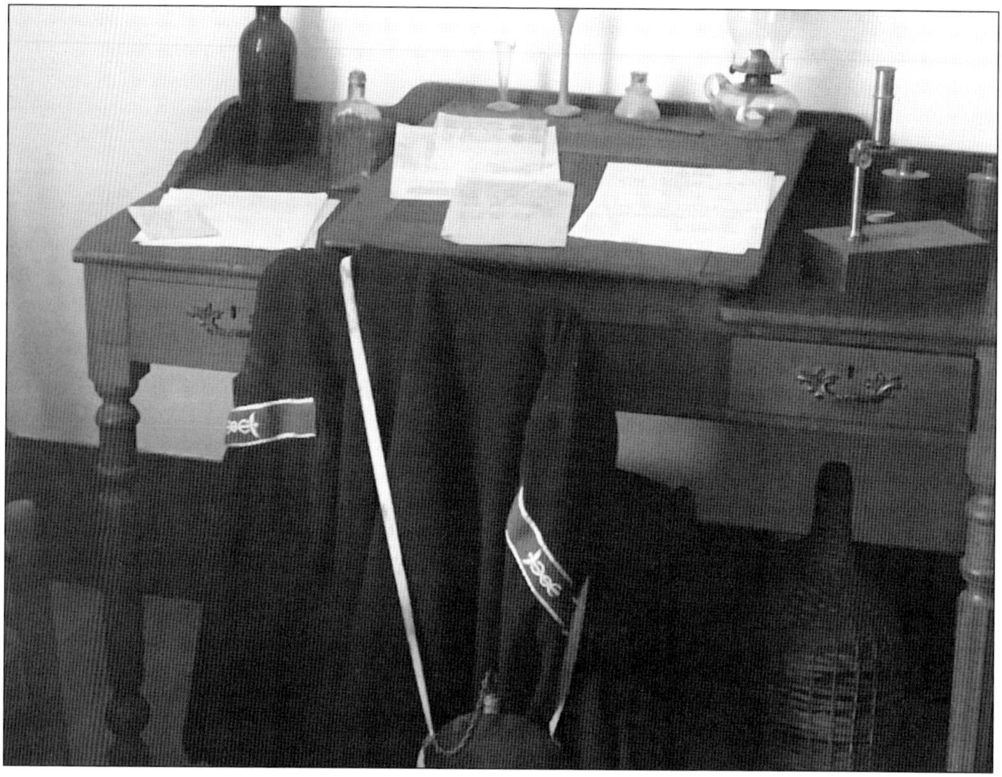

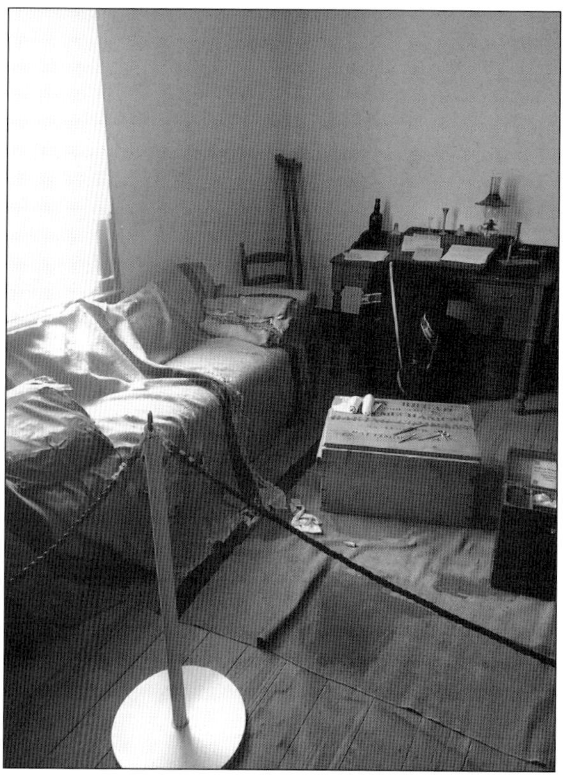

An interior view of the Harper House is seen above along with a recreation of how a Union medical officer's desk might appear from the period. The battle spanned from March 19 to March 21, 1865, with more than 500 injured soldiers being cared for in the house and tents surrounding the home. Sherman reunited his army of more than 50,000 men and overpowered the Confederates. Johnston withdrew March 21, and Sherman moved on to Goldsboro, taking his wounded with him.

Another interior view of the Harper House includes bandages, pharmaceutical, and surgical equipment. The floor shows actual blood stains from the dozens of surgeries known to have been performed in this specific area during and after the Bentonville battle.

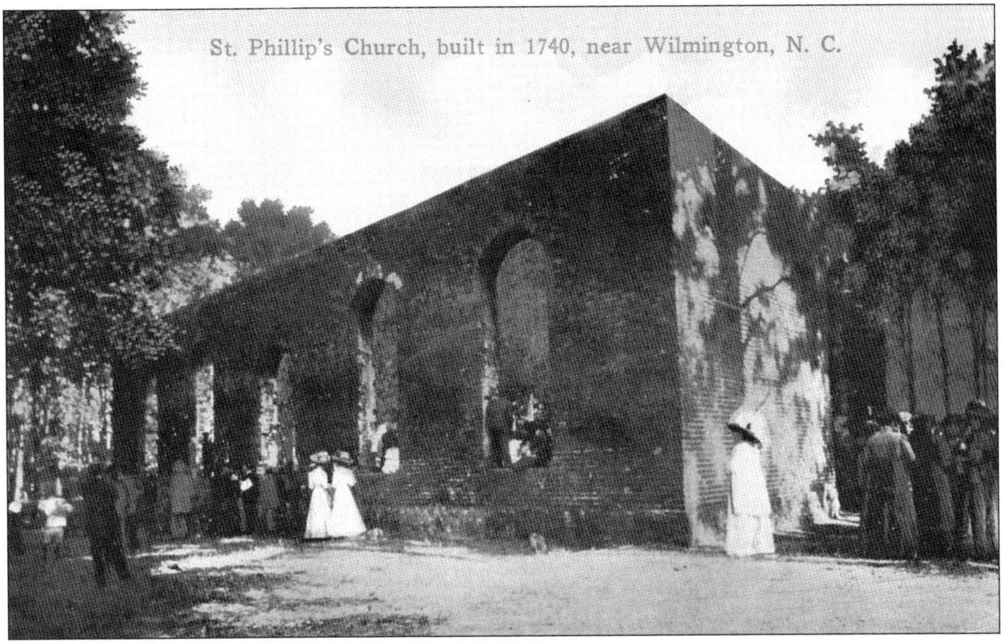

Following the February 1865 Confederate evacuation of Forts Johnston and Anderson, the St. Phillips Church, in old Brunswick Town, was seized and occupied by the Union army. It was used as a hospital for their wounded. Fort Anderson was a small earthworks fort across the Cape Fear River from Fort Fisher and just north of Fort Johnston. Located near Orton Plantation and St. Phillips Church, it was identified as the "Quarantine Fort" on a February 1865 map published in the *Illustrated London News*. In addition to the hospital at St. Phillips Church, Union troops used the main house at Orton Plantation for smallpox cases.

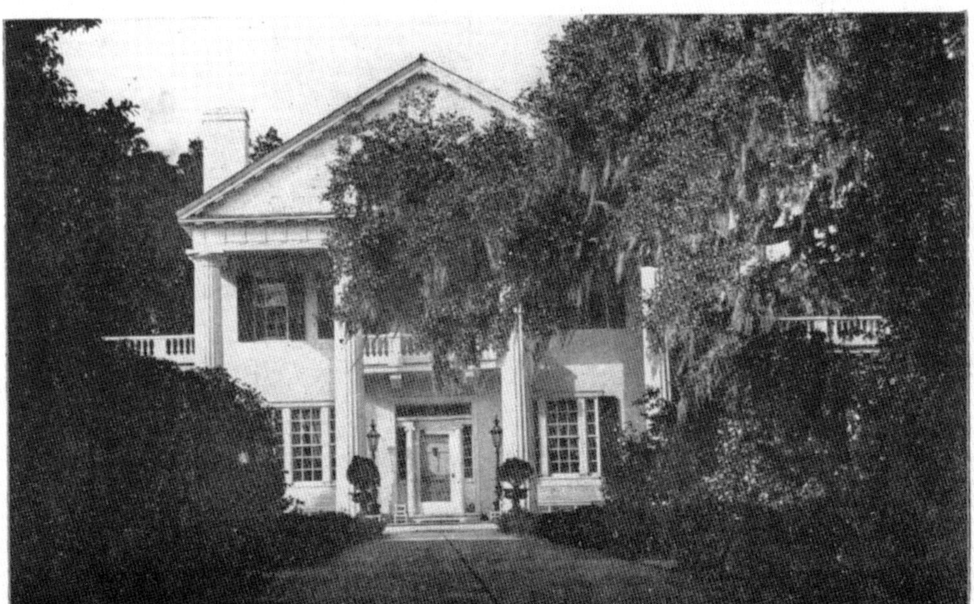

BEAUTIFUL ORTON MANSION, ON ORTON PLANTATION, NEAR SOUTHPORT, N. C.

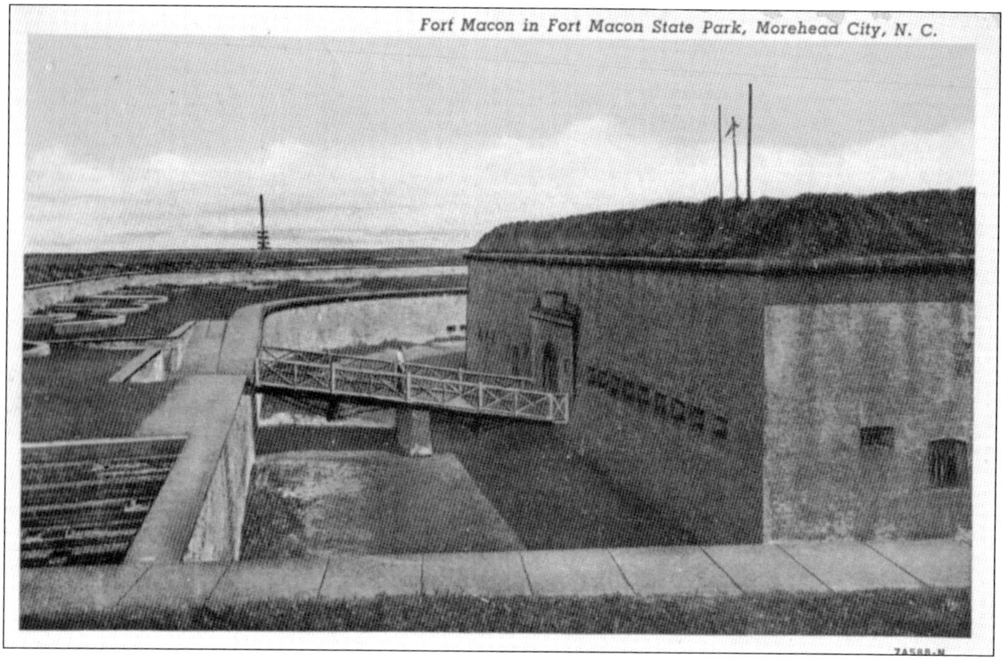
Fort Macon in Fort Macon State Park, Morehead City, N. C.

Construction began on Fort Macon in Carteret County in 1826. While garrisons of soldiers would occasionally man the fort, it was mostly abandoned until being seized by North Carolina militia in April 1861 representing the Confederate government. Union forces would recapture the fort following a two-day bombardment in April 1862.

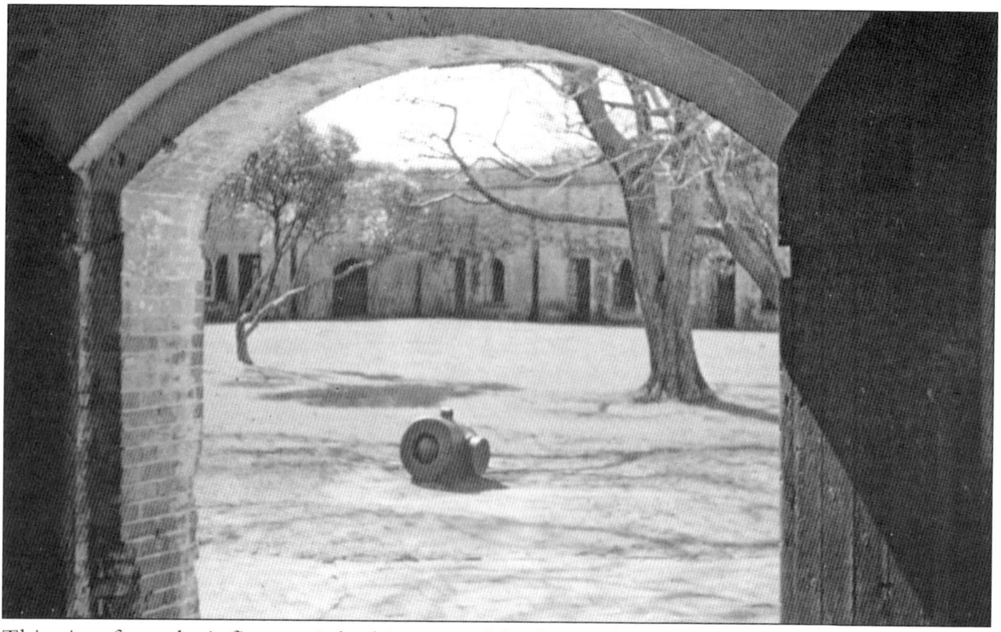

This view from the infirmary is looking out of the fort at the interior of Fort Macon's grounds. By 1870, a salvaged building was being used as a makeshift hospital. A report by the post surgeon, Dr. Elliott Coues, stated, "The hospital is a disgrace to the service." He goes on to describe the dereliction of the building and concludes with, "no possible repairs will fit the building for hospital purposes. The absolute and pressing necessity for a new hospital is obvious."

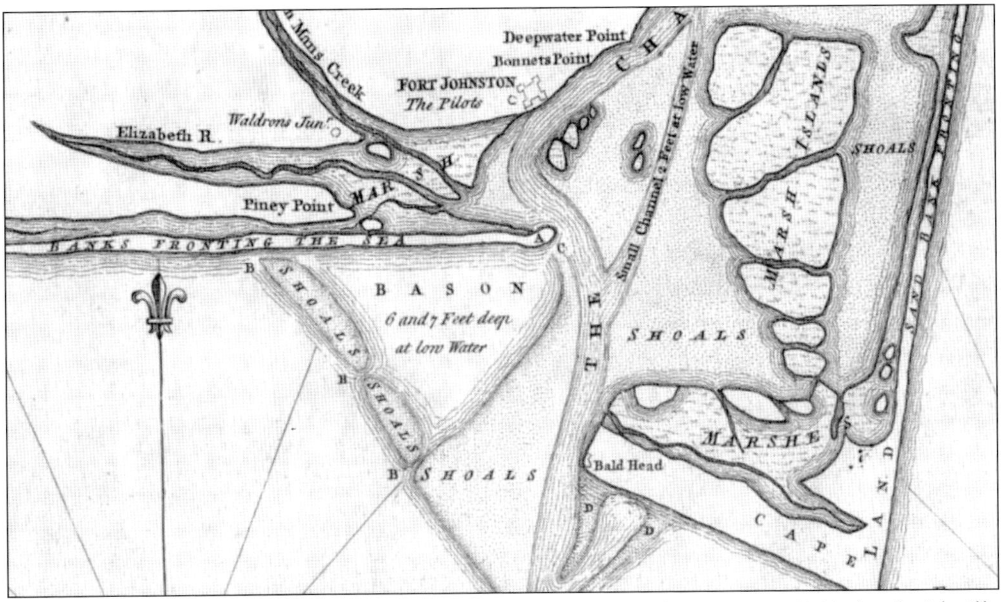

Construction began on Governor Johnston's fort, Fort Johnston, in 1748 in Smithville (Southport). It was designated as a quarantine station for vessels arriving at the port in 1751. Colonists burned the fort in 1775. A rebuilt fort (over the ruins of the old structure) was completed in 1816 to include "a battery of eight guns, a blockhouse, a guardhouse, a hospital, and buildings for enlisted as well as officers' quarters." (Southport Historical Society, 1749 Hyrne map.)

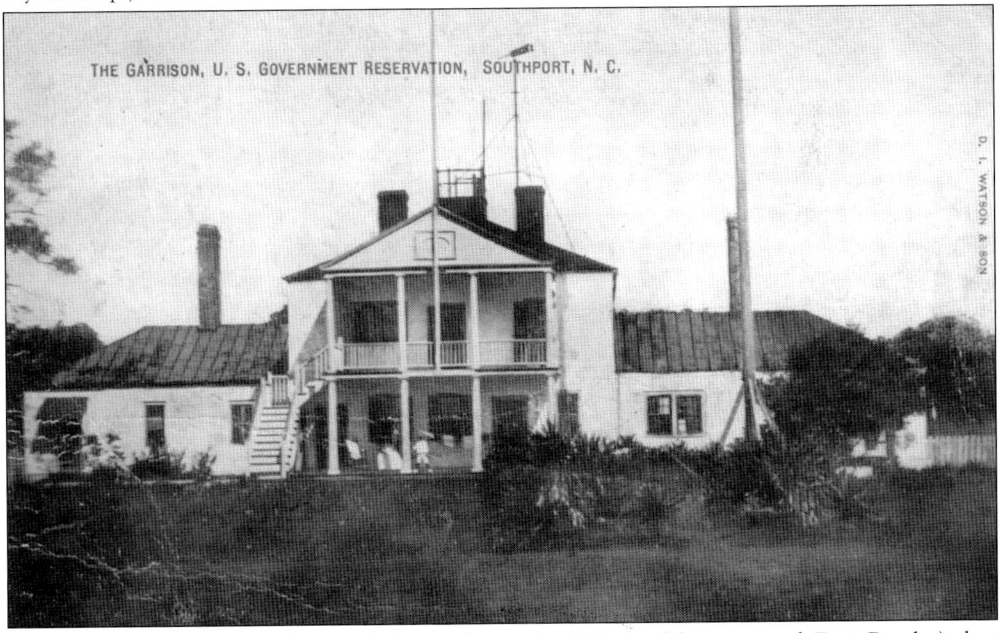
THE GARRISON, U. S. GOVERNMENT RESERVATION, SOUTHPORT, N. C.
D. I. WATSON & SON

Fort Johnston was seized by Confederate forces in 1861 (and later named Fort Pender), but when Fort Fisher fell in 1865, the Confederates abandoned the remaining defensive forts in the region. Pictured here from an early-1900s postcard, the Garrison House was restored in the 1890s for use by the US Signal Service. Today, the historical structure is operated as the North Carolina Maritime Museum.

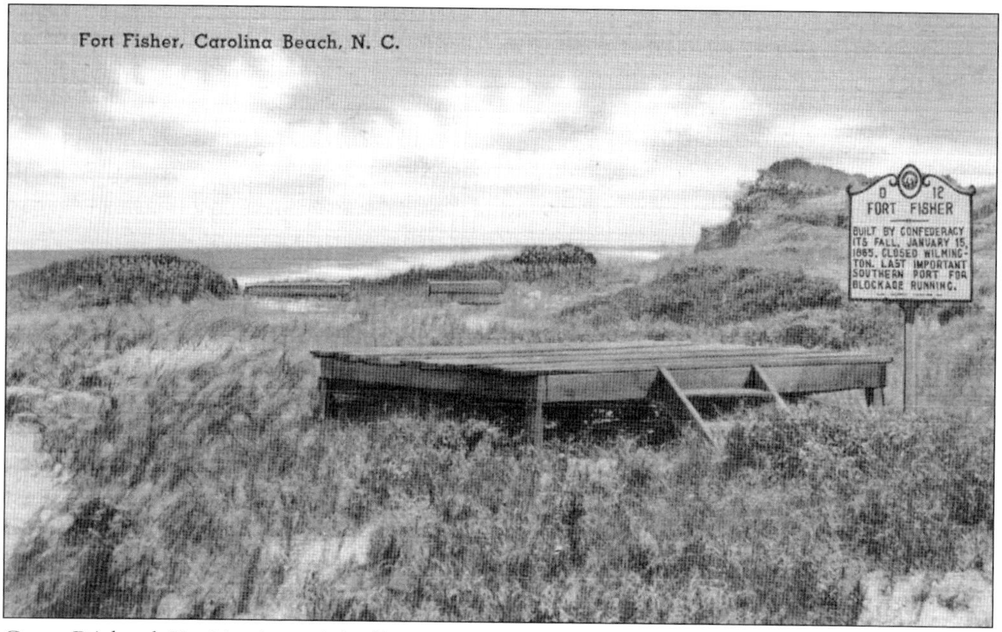
Fort Fisher, Carolina Beach, N. C.
D 12
FORT FISHER
BUILT BY CONFEDERACY
ITS FALL, JANUARY 15,
1865, CLOSED WILMING-
TON, LAST IMPORTANT
SOUTHERN PORT FOR
BLOCKADE RUNNING.

Capt. Richard K. Meade, originally a Union engineer and officer at Fort Sumter before resigning his commission, arrived at Fort Fisher as a Confederate engineer during the summer of 1861. Shortly thereafter, he began construction of Hospital Battery Meade. Colonel Lamb would later bombproof the structure, creating the post hospital.

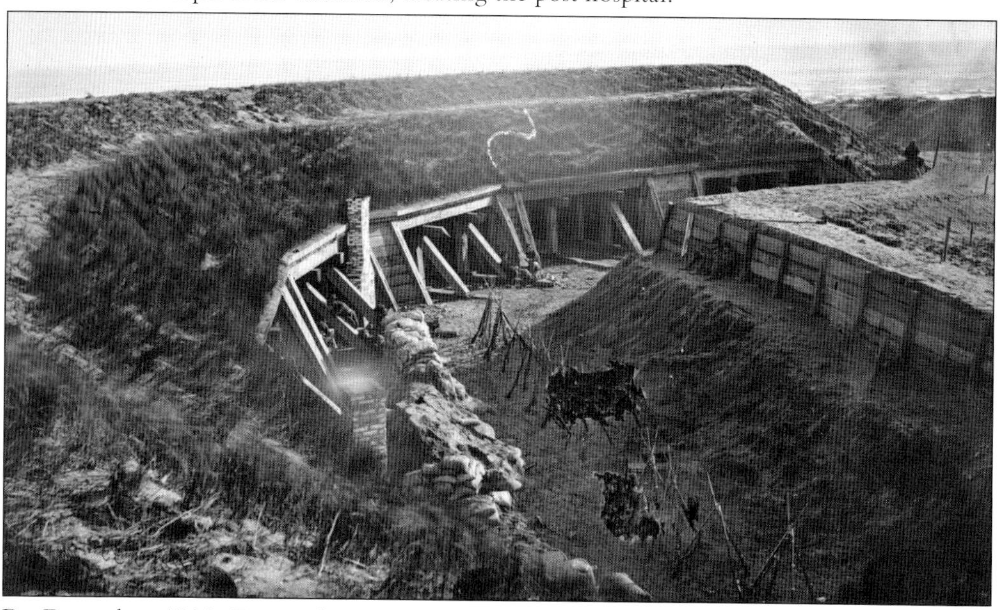

By December 1864, Fort Fisher was an immense earthwork and the world's largest fort. However, an equally formidable force of 64 Union warships had amassed for an attack. On Christmas Eve, Union warships fired 20,271 shells at the massive fort. Hospital Battery Meade saw limited casualties after this assault, as the Union was unable to defeat the Confederates. The Confederate win was short-lived, as thousands of Union Marines came ashore north of the fort and overran the Confederate position on January 15, 1865. (Image LC-B8171-7535, Library of Congress.)

Six

Military and Veterans Hospitals

Multiple forts in Eastern North Carolina were created or expanded during the great world wars. These locations included Fort Bragg (Fayetteville) and Camp Lejeune (Jacksonville). Other locations included the Coast Guard Station (Elizabeth City), the Army Air Field Seymour Johnson (Goldsboro), as well as Pope Army Air Field, adjacent to Fort Bragg. Naval Air Station Cherry Point was also located just south of Camp Lejeune. Other historical locations included Camp Davis (between Wilmington and Camp Lejeune) as well as reactivating historical Forts Macon and Caswell, where soldiers were stationed and trained.

Eastern North Carolina offered an ideal location for injured troops to recover based on ease of access once returning from Europe. As the Veterans Administration began to construct hospitals, Fayetteville was a logical location based on the sizable military presence in the region.

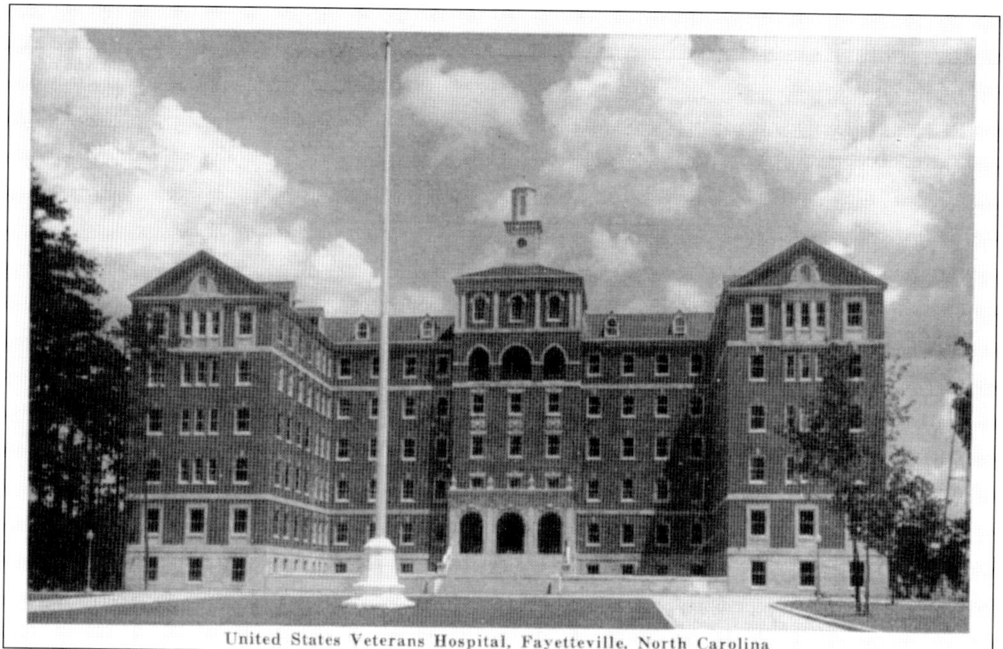

Between 1930 and 1945, the number of Veterans Administration hospitals doubled from 45 to 97, including a new one approximately 10 miles from Fort Bragg. It opened in 1939 at 2300 Ramsey Street.

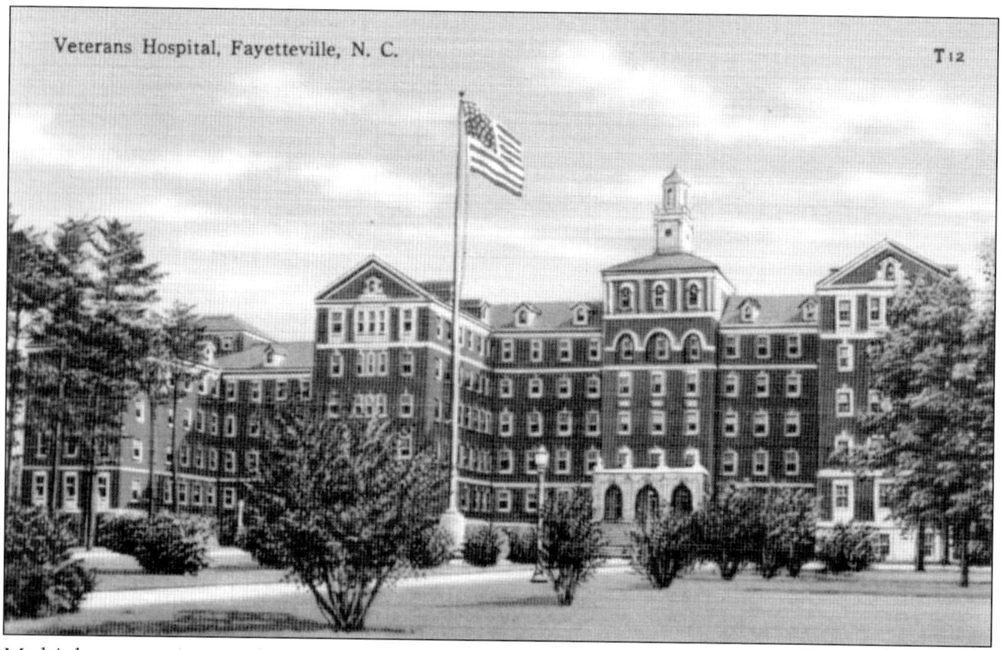

Multiple renovations and additions have taken place through the years. Included in the picture is a four-story wing that was added to the east side of the facility in the early 1950s.

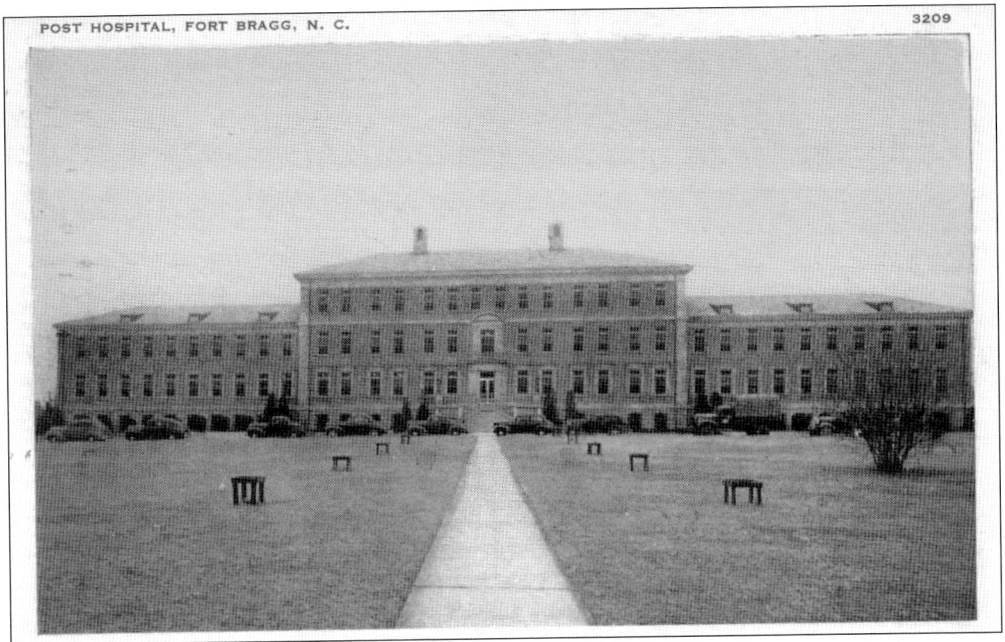

The Fort Bragg Post Hospital (pictured here in the early 1930s) was an 83-bed, three-story hospital. It replaced the Camp Bragg Base Hospital, a series of 22 building with a capacity of 500 beds. Today, this building is the headquarters for the XVIII Airborne Corps.

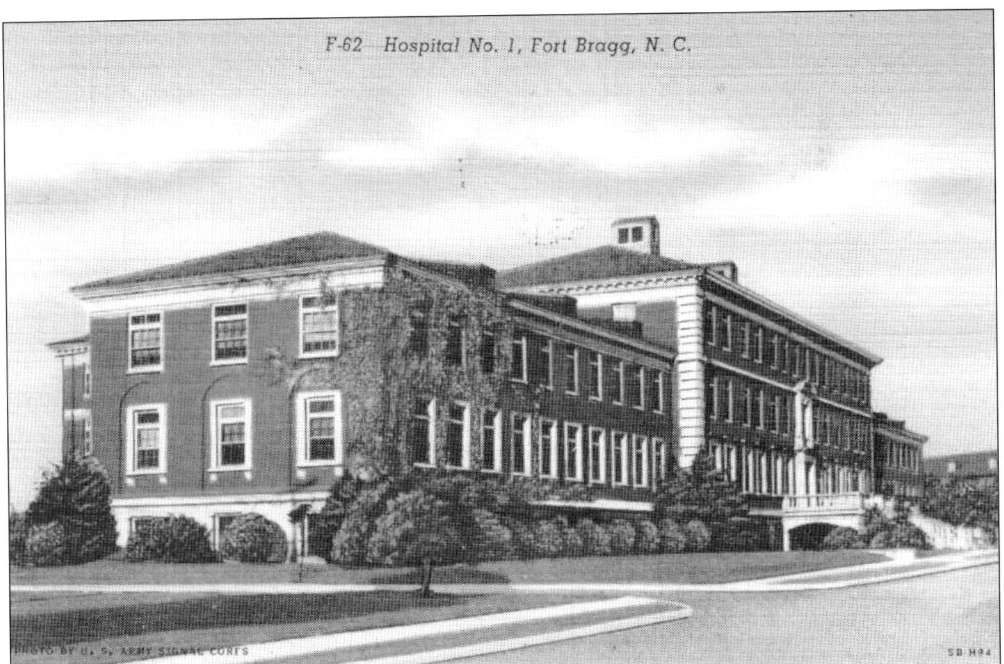

Previously referred to as the "Post Hospital," the hospital became known as USA Station Hospital One. By 1941, the hospital would be replaced by USA Station Hospitals Two and Three, and the building was converted into a headquarters for XVIII Airborne Troops.

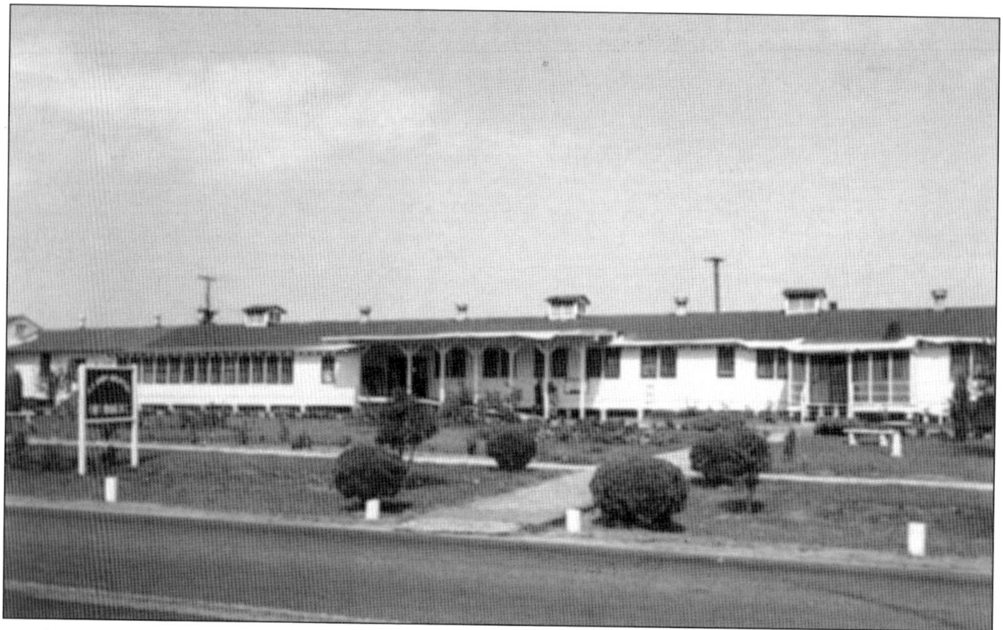

At the corner of Reilly and Normandy Roads is the street-side view of the main entrance of the USA Station Hospital at Fort Bragg. The station hospitals were placed under one command in 1942. Most of the hospital facilities quickly closed after the end of World War II. The station hospital services consolidated into this facility for the next 10 years until being replaced by Womack Army Community Hospital.

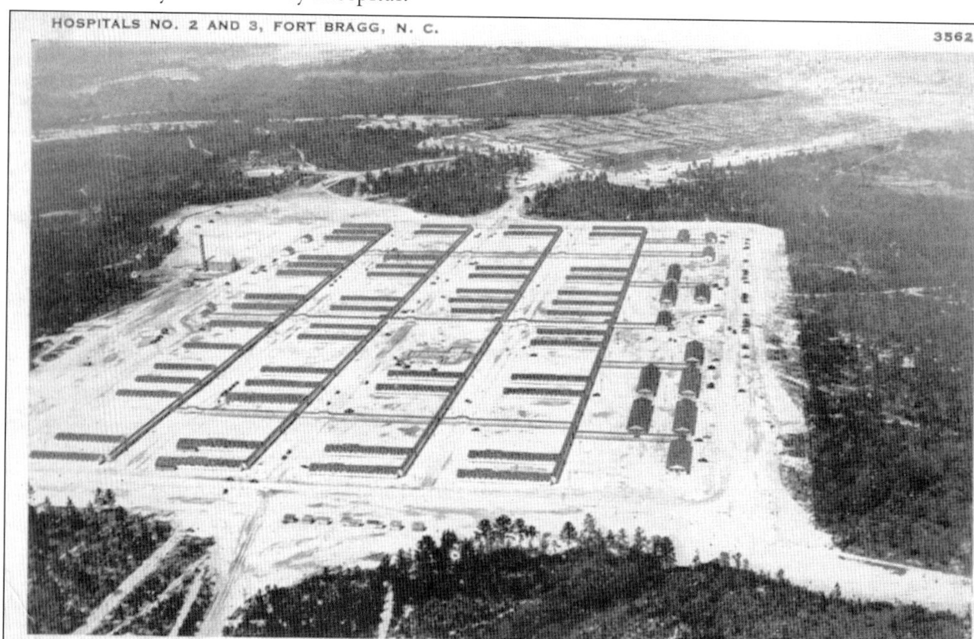

In February 1941, two cantonment-type hospitals, also known as USA Station Hospitals Two and Three, were built to accommodate patients from the war raging in Europe. By May 1941, the bed capacity was 2,682. Additional capacity was created by using the buildings of the Infantry Brigade of the Ninth Division as USA Station Hospital Four.

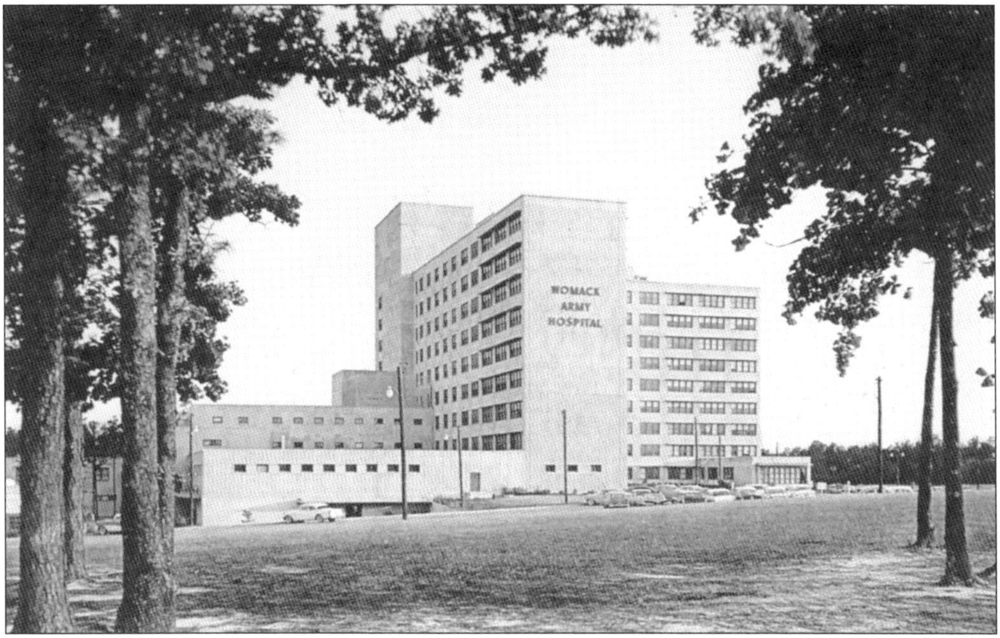

In May 1955, construction began on the Womack Army Community Hospital to replace the USA Station Hospital. It was named for Army medic and North Carolina native Pfc. Bryant Homer Womack, who was posthumously awarded the Congressional Medal of Honor for his actions in Korea. The nine-story, 500-bed hospital opened on August 3, 1958. A replacement hospital (Womack Army Medical Center) opened at 2817 Riley Road in March 2000.

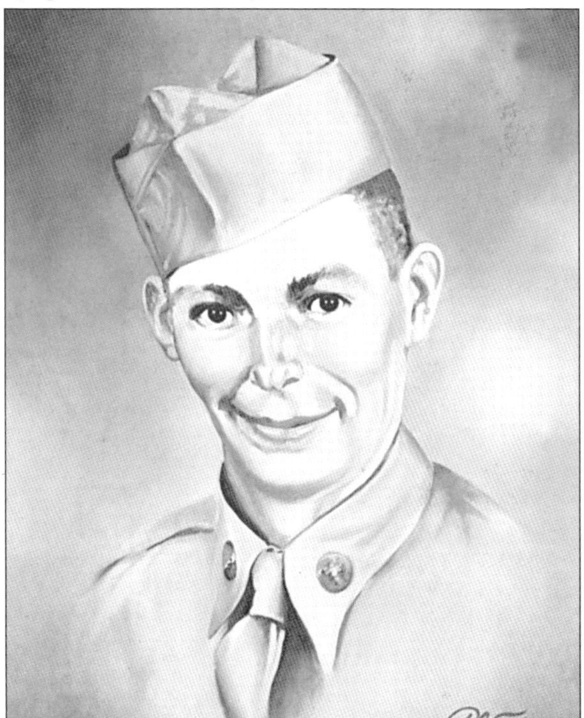

Pfc. Bryant Homer Womack and his unit came under heavy enemy fire on March 12, 1952, in Korea. Throughout the night, Womack provided aid and directed care even after losing his arm following a mortar explosion. He was the last man to withdraw but later died from blood loss. He was posthumously awarded the Congressional Medal of Honor. (Office of Medical History, Army Medical Department Regiment.)

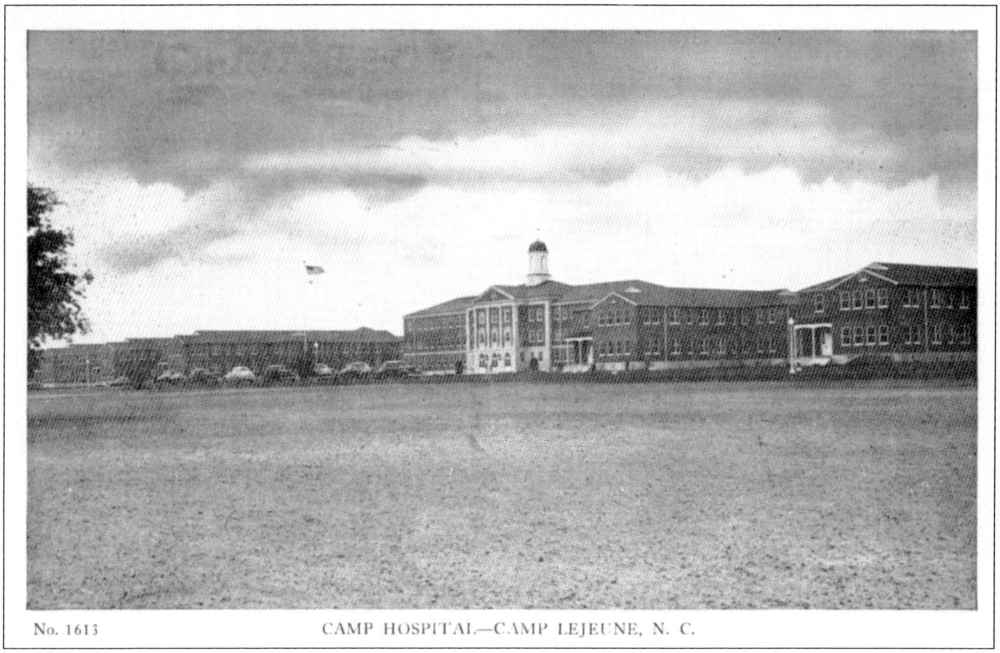
No. 1613
CAMP HOSPITAL—CAMP LEJEUNE, N. C.

In February 1941, the US Navy received approval to construct a training center near Jacksonville, later named Camp Lejeune. The Hadnot Point peninsula was selected for the original hospital (pictured above) in 1942. The US Naval Hospital Jacksonville officially opened on May 1, 1943. With both water and air access, the hospital was a convenient stop for US Navy ships evacuating wounded marines and sailors from Europe.

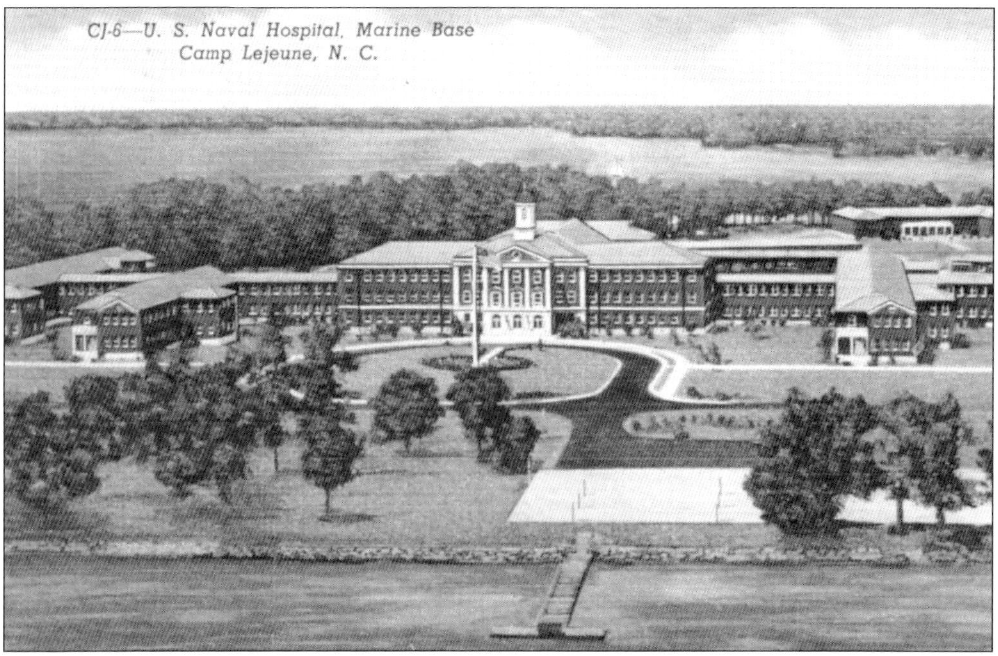
CJ-6—U. S. Naval Hospital, Marine Base
Camp Lejeune, N. C.

Another view (port side) of the original Camp Lejeune Naval Hospital is pictured above. At its peak during World War II, there were approximately 2,100 patients in the hospital. The hospital continued to serve the US Marine Corps with distinction until being replaced 1983.

While the previous photographs offer a view of the central hospital buildings, most images belie the enormous complex constructed on the Hadnot Point peninsula. This aerial image offers a more comprehensive view of the resources for the medical center and the military post. In keeping with traditional Navy hospital construction, the facility was buffered from the noise and well away from other activities to minimize the spread of contagions.

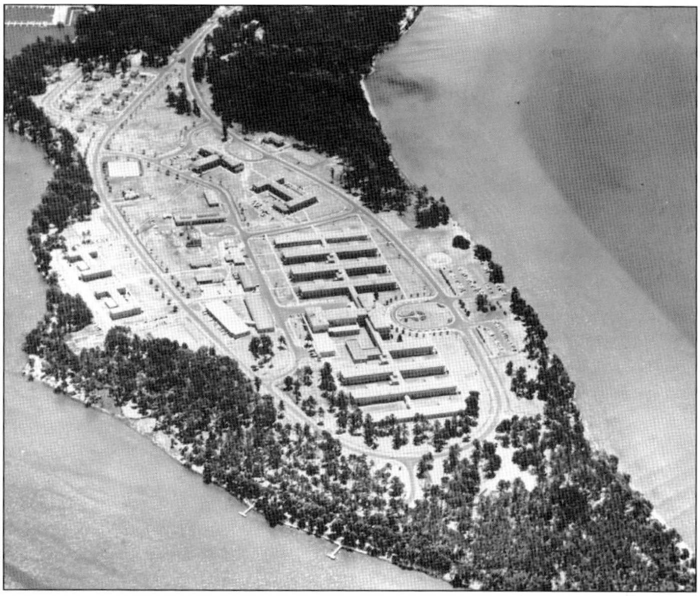

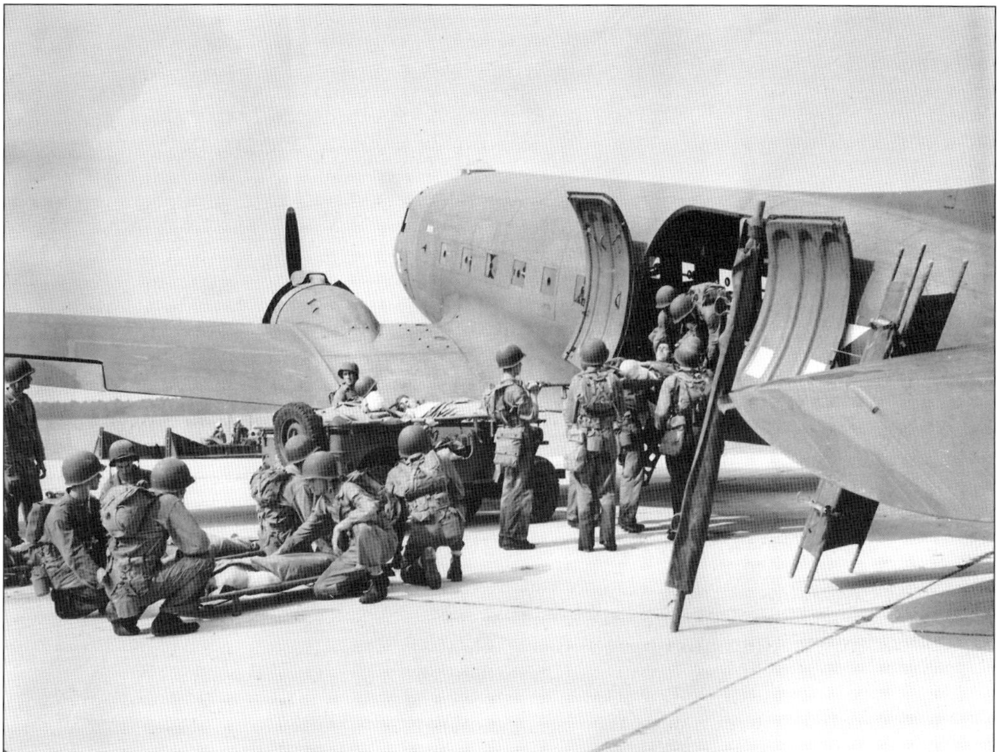

This photograph from July 15, 1943, highlights a simulated attack on an enemy-held island near the port access to Camp Lejeune. The exercise reflects the role medical corpsmen play during an attack. This simulated attack included air, ground, and sea assault and tested the importance of rapid evacuation from a battlefield by air and sea, eventually ship to shore (in this case, the naval hospital at Camp Lejeune).

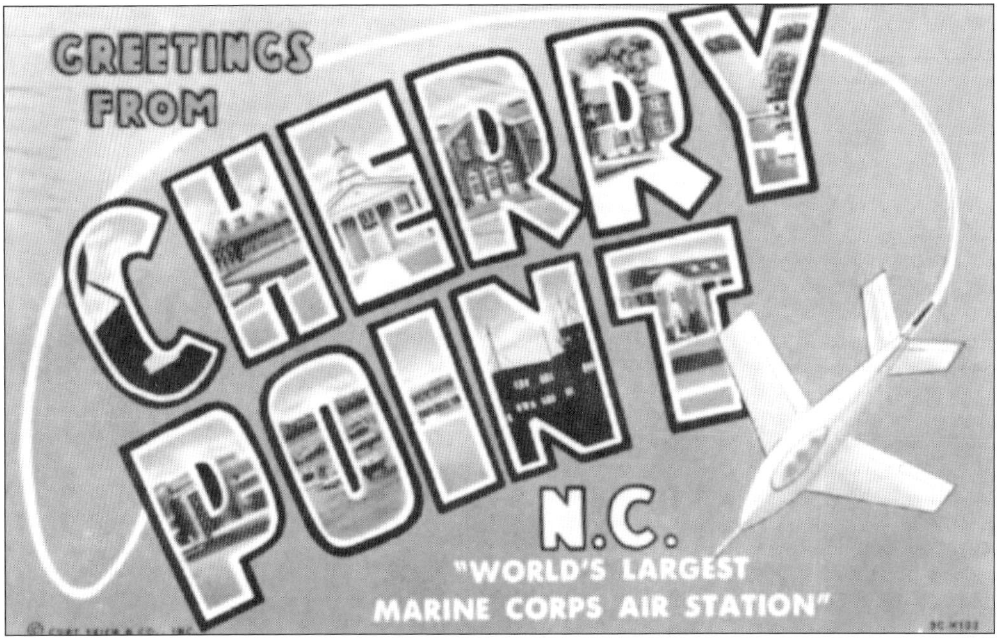

The US Marine Corps Air Station Hospital at Cherry Point (Craven County) was established in 1943 as a general dispensary (hospital). By 1956, it was reported to have 70 beds and 22 bassinets. The dispensary was commissioned as a naval hospital July 1, 1968. A new hospital was built and opened on October 1, 1994. By 2007, the hospital transitioned to an outpatient clinic.

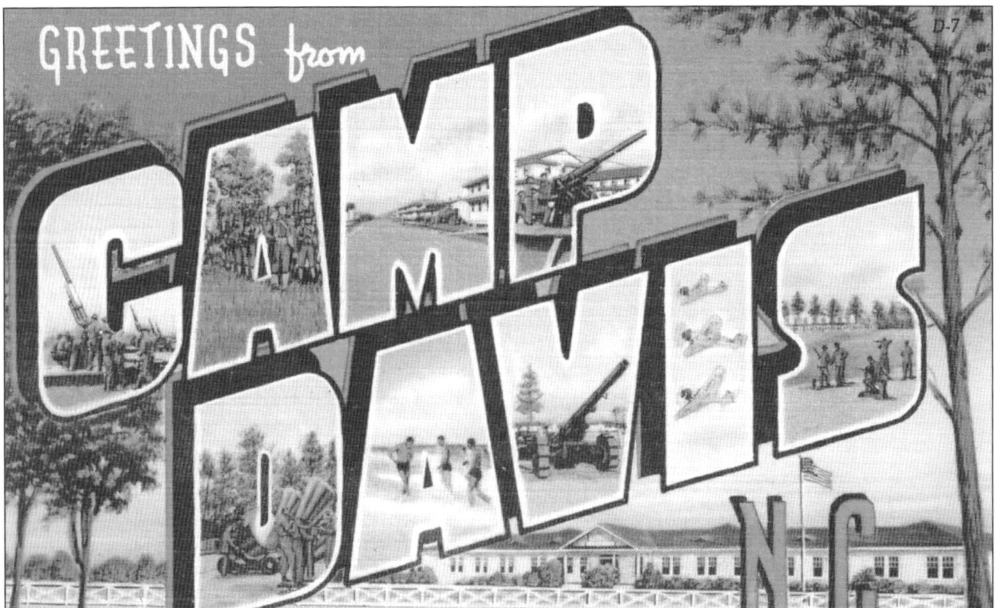

By early 1941, major construction was under way creating a new antiaircraft artillery training center near the town of Holly Ridge, in Onslow County, to be called Camp Davis. The base included an 800-bed hospital. In 1946, the Army Air Force briefly used it as a convalescent center. By the late 1940s, the base was dismantled. The runways today are used by the US Marines for the V22 Osprey program.

Seven

Temporary Hospitals

From war to disease outbreaks and disasters, adapted spaces such as churches and schools, augmented by tents, have been used for centuries as temporary hospitals. Worldwide, the 1918 influenza pandemic death totals rivaled that of both world wars combined. The flu came to North Carolina in September 1918 and quickly overwhelmed the hospitals. The pandemic was caused by a novel influenza virus that spread worldwide, leaving tens of millions ill and millions more dead. A standard solution during the pandemic included the use of temporary hospitals.

In the 1950s, the Cold War and the threat of thermonuclear war with the Soviet Union resulted in a bolstering of civil defense and preparedness. One provision of civil defense included the creation of multiple temporary hospital packages (Civil Defense Emergency Hospitals), which were stationed around North Carolina.

In the aftermath of the September 11, 2001, attacks, multiple temporary hospitals were created in various states to bolster bed capacity in the aftermath of a disaster. These resources have since been used for several disaster responses, such as Hurricanes Katrina and Matthew.

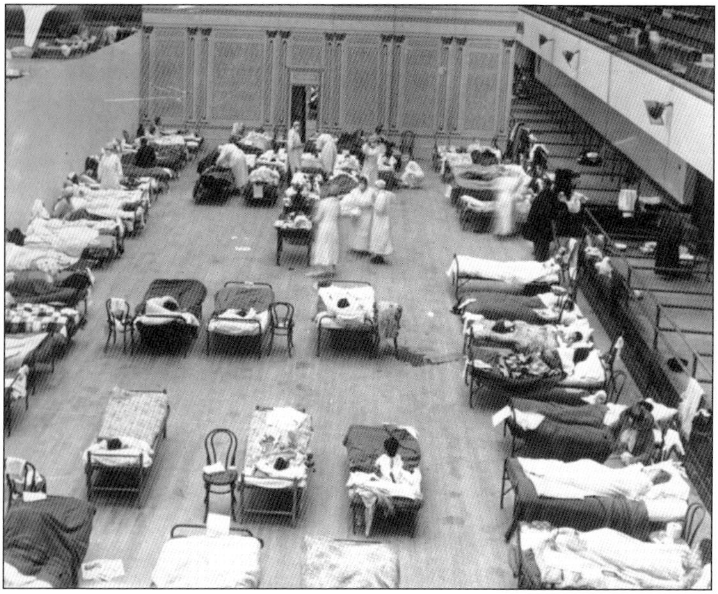

A report to the North Carolina State Board of Health in 1918 noted that "all the hospitals are crowded" and that the disease was "epidemic" in several cities. This 1918 US Public Health photograph from Oakland, California, reveals the common layout when churches and schools were used as emergency hospitals in cities such as Charlotte, Raleigh, Rocky Mount, Wilmington, and Fayetteville.

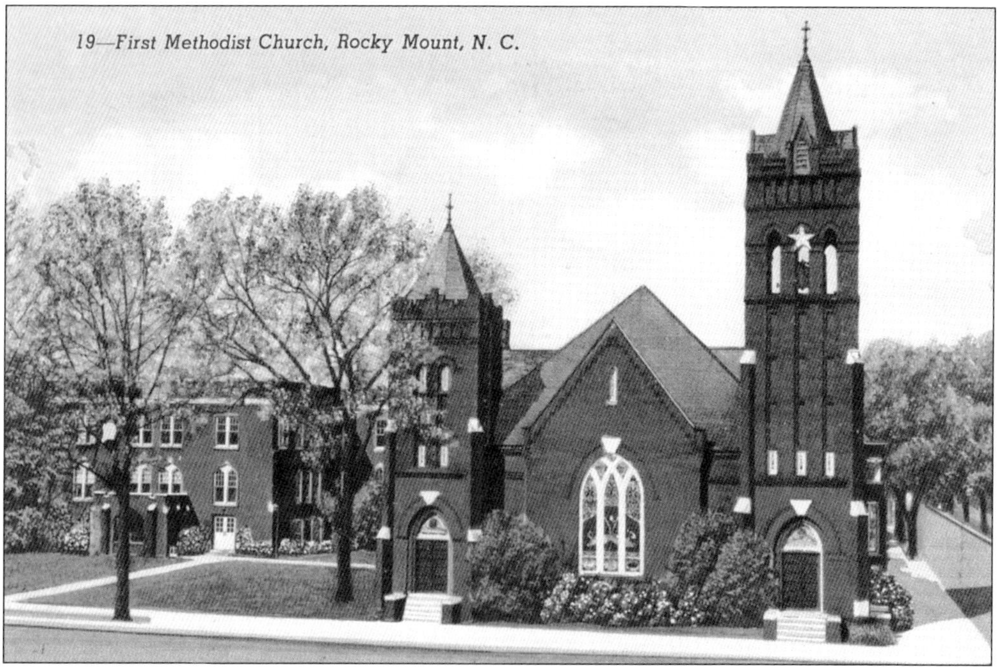

First Methodist Church, Rocky Mount was the home of an emergency hospital during the 1918 flu pandemic. Across North Carolina, more than 100,000 fell ill and another 13,703 died between October 1918 and March 1919. The pandemic was also marked by a rather unsophisticated response where little other than supportive care could be offered. However, it appears that merely placing sick patients in sequestered medical facilities decreased the spread of disease.

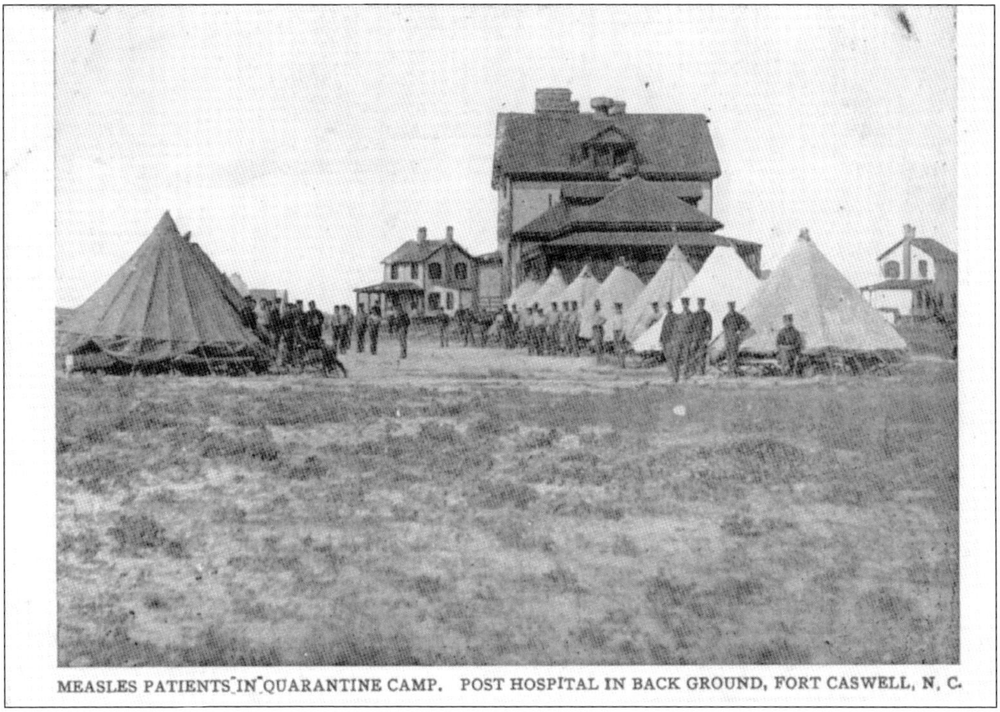
MEASLES PATIENTS IN QUARANTINE CAMP. POST HOSPITAL IN BACK GROUND, FORT CASWELL, N. C.

On December 17, 1917, the *Charlotte Observer* reported a severe measles outbreak at Fort Caswell in Brunswick County. A quarantine camp surrounding the post hospital was established at the fort.

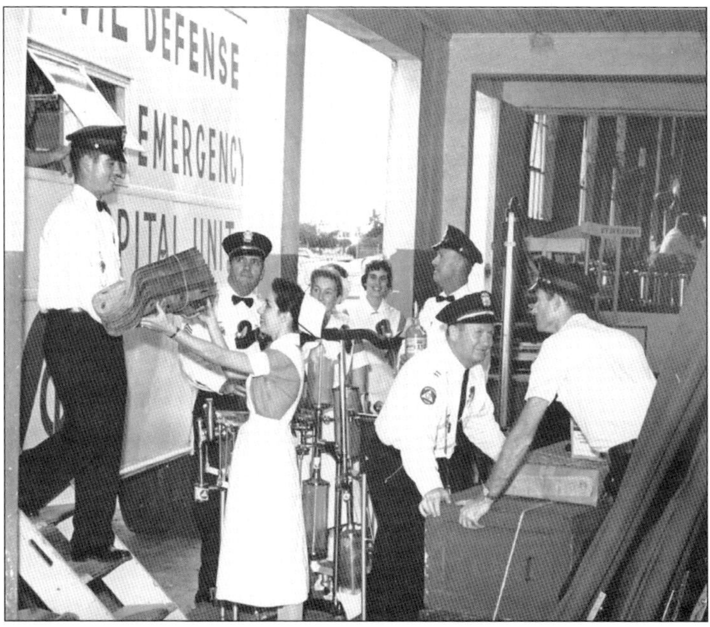
DEFENSE

In the aftermath of World War II, tensions rose quickly between the United States and the United Soviet Socialist Republic (USSR). In the United States, the civilian defense programs began to prepare for the new and looming threat of a thermonuclear attack by the USSR. One of the components of the civil defense program included creating the Civil Defense Emergency Hospitals (CDEH).

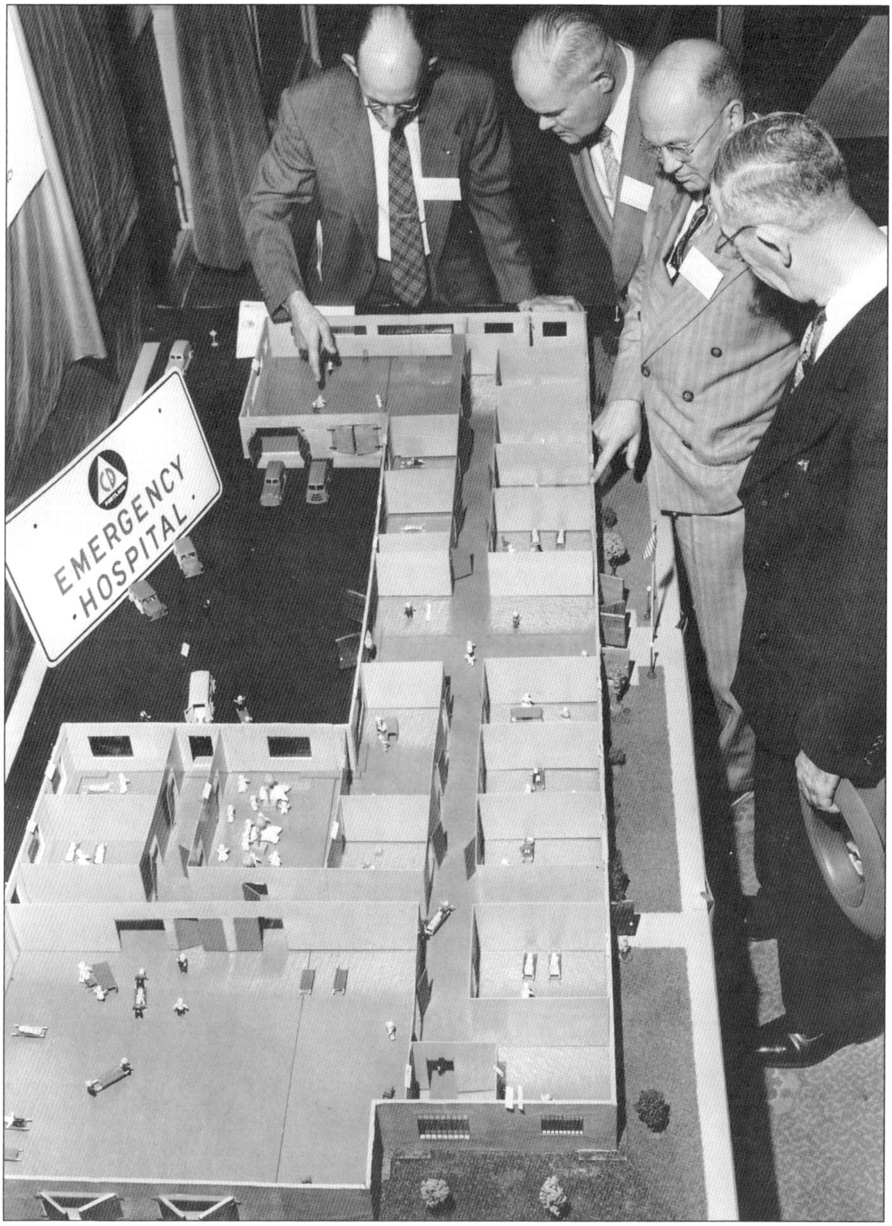

Shown here is a CDEH mock-up on display; the setting is a school building. The CDEH included medical supplies and equipment sufficient for up to 30 days of operation, 200 stretchers, oxygen, an operating room, a pharmacy, and X-ray and laboratory equipment. The CDEH relied on adapted space in a community building, school, or church. Local medical personnel and volunteers would staff these temporary facilities, which were created to deal with the expected surge of casualties. With the close of the Vietnam conflict, two US economic recessions, and a general shift in priorities, much of the federal support dissolved for the civil defense program. By the late 1970s, most of the CDEHs had been abandoned or the materials scavenged for use by local hospitals and the emerging emergency medical service (EMS) agencies. At the height of the program, the CDEHs were distributed around the country, with 35 located across North Carolina.

Pictured is an armband worn by CDEH medical personnel. Frequently associated with the CDEH, the white pyramid on the blue background was and remains a standard emblem of emergency management.

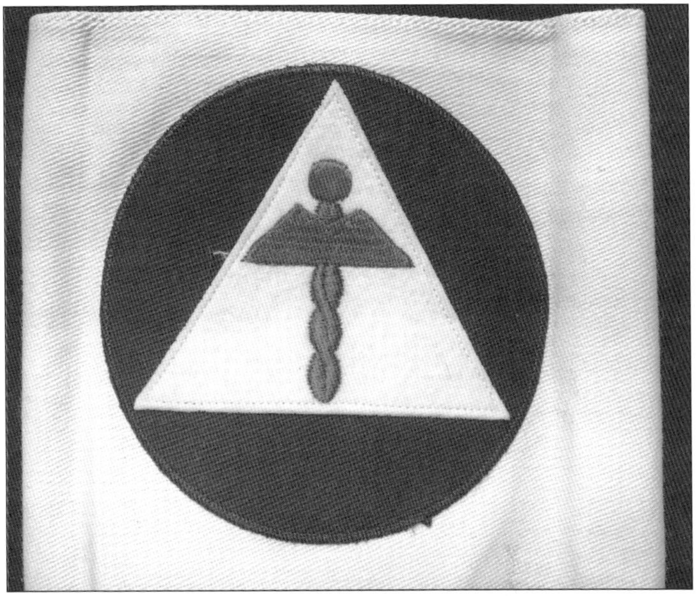

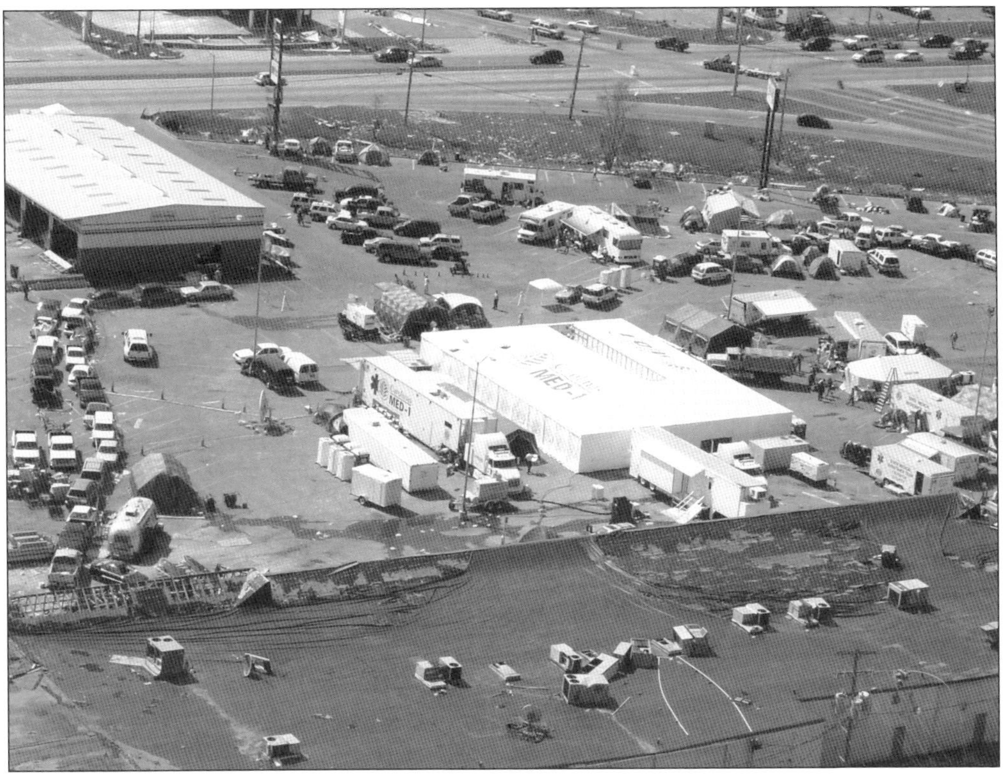

In the aftermath of Hurricane Katrina, the State Medical Assistance Team (SMAT), including teams from multiple hospitals in Eastern North Carolina, along with MED-1 from Carolinas Medical Center, responded to Waveland, Mississippi. The response supported a hospital that was damaged by the hurricane (Hancock Regional Medical Center). The SMAT hospital operated in September and October 2005. During that time, 7,500 patients were treated and another 15,000 needed vaccinations or replacement prescriptions.

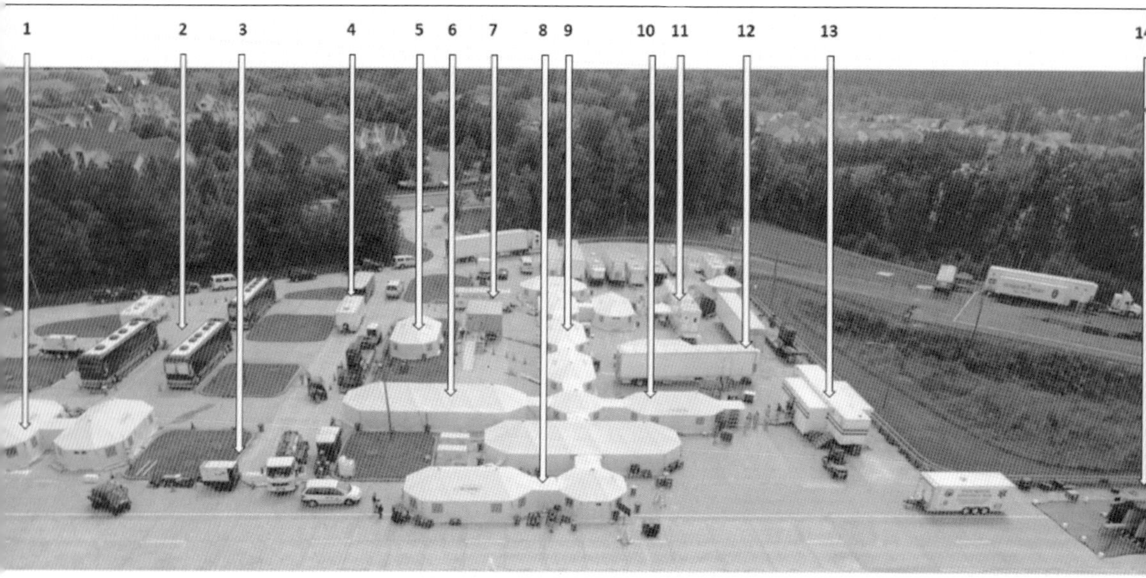

The North Carolina SMAT Field Hospital, 2012.

This layout features components of the National Mobile Disaster Hospital connected with components of the State Medical Support Shelter and other state/federal agencies.

1-Crew quarters, meeting area. 2-DMAT Crew Buses. 3-Generator. 4-Crew Quarters Western Shelter Support. 5-Command. 6-MDH Critical Care Unit. 7-MDH X-ray. 8-Emergency Department and Triage. 9-SMSS patient care areas. 10-Surgical Processing. 11-SMAT Crew Quarters & Observation Deck. 12-Supply Trailer. 13-MDH Mobile Operating Rooms. 14-Decontamination Tent

Shown here is a more complete build out of one of the SMAT hospitals, fully mobilized during the 2012 Democratic National Convention held in Charlotte. This temporary hospital was designed to absorb additional patients in the event of a mass casualty event. Supplemental aid stations were positioned around the city near the convention center, detention center, football stadium, and entry checkpoints for the secure areas of the convention. This hospital can accommodate up to 400 patients, with two operating rooms and typical supporting services for 100-plus medical personnel and staff.

Eight

General Hospitals

The American Medical Association began publishing the American Medical Directory in 1906 to completely catalog the hospitals, sanatoriums, and related institutions for each state and US territory, which at the time included the Canal Zone and the Philippine Islands. (This rather massive book also included all medical schools and all physicians in each state.)

By 1950, the 18th edition of the American Medical Directory reported 166 hospitals, sanatoriums, and related institutions in North Carolina. There were 46 hospitals in the Eastern North Carolina region at the time. Just two years later, the 19th edition reported 189 hospitals, sanatoriums, and related institutions with 57 in the region. This chapter will explore many of the institutions during the 20th century. Some have grown, and some have closed.

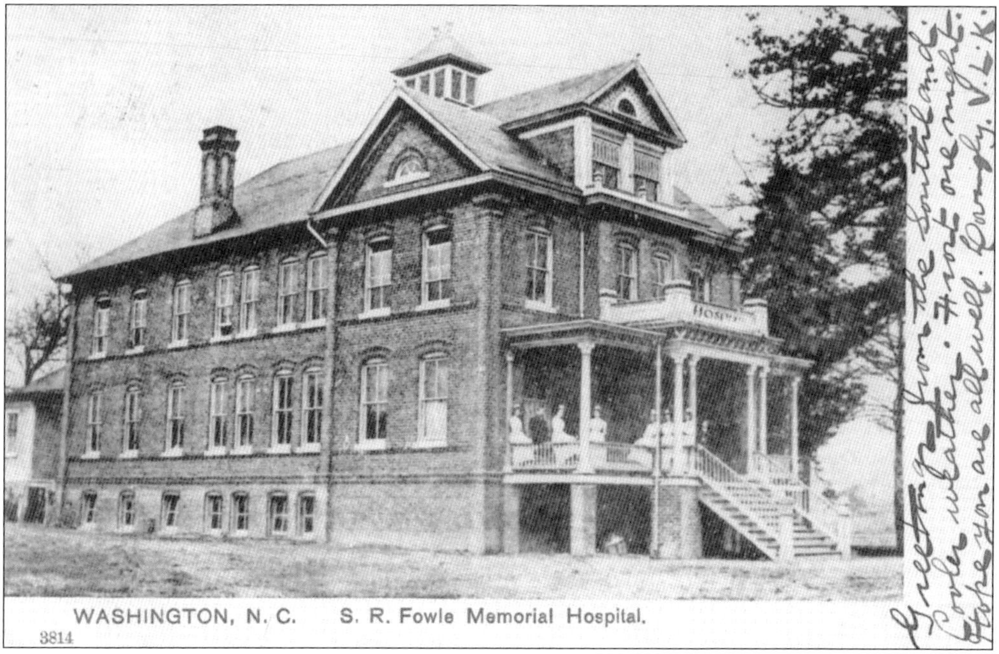

The S.R. Fowle Memorial Hospital was established in 1903 (or 1904, sources vary). By 1923, Dr. John L. Nicholson operated the 30-bed hospital. The hospital closed when Beaufort County Hospital opened in 1958. The building was located at Fifth and Market Streets but later was demolished and replaced by the Washington Fire Department.

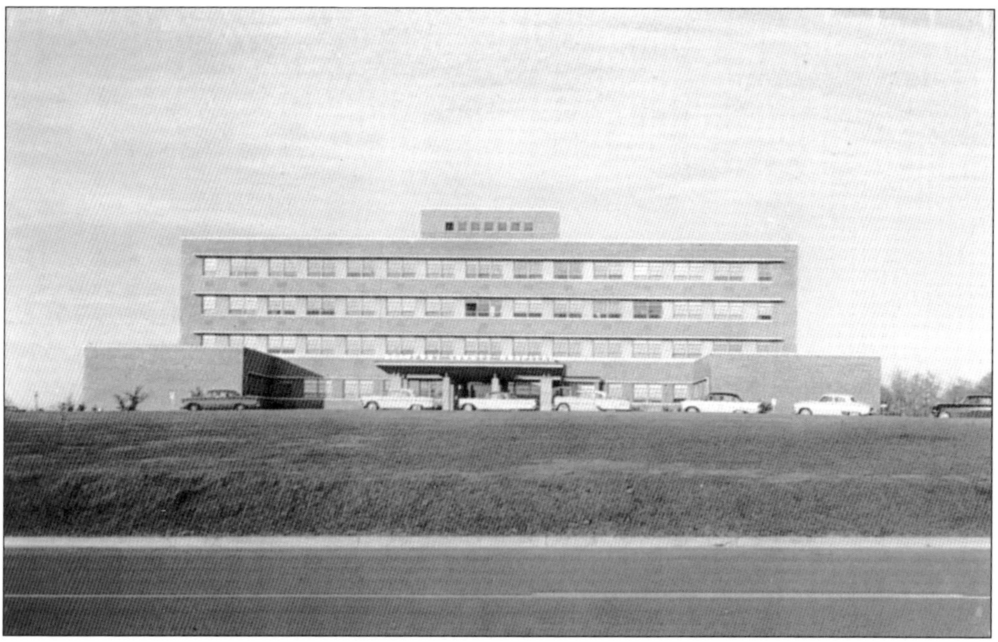

Beaufort County Hospital opened in 1958, financed in part by Hill-Burton funds; the new consolidated hospital replaced the remaining Washington area hospitals. Located at 628 East Twelfth Street, today this hospital is known as Vidant Beaufort Hospital.

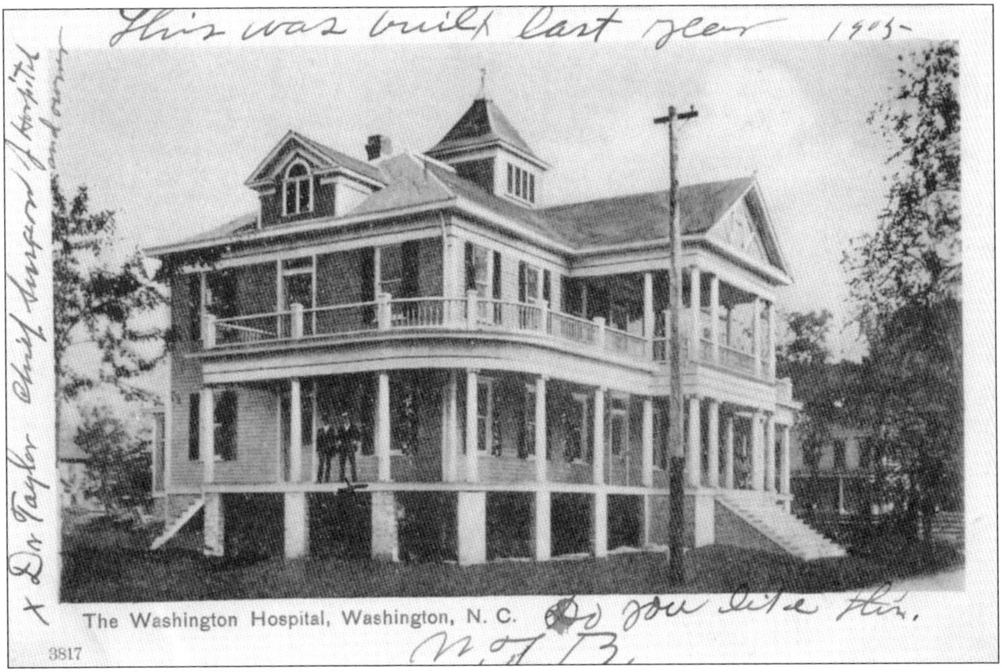
This was built last year 1905
The Washington Hospital, Washington, N. C.
Do you like this.
3817

The Washington Hospital was established in 1904 (also known as the River View/Riverview Hospital) in Beaufort County. Dr. D.T. Tayloe (pictured on the porch here) operated the 35-bed hospital. He later purchased the private hospital, adding to the building and renaming it the Tayloe Hospital. It closed when the Beaufort County Hospital opened in 1958.

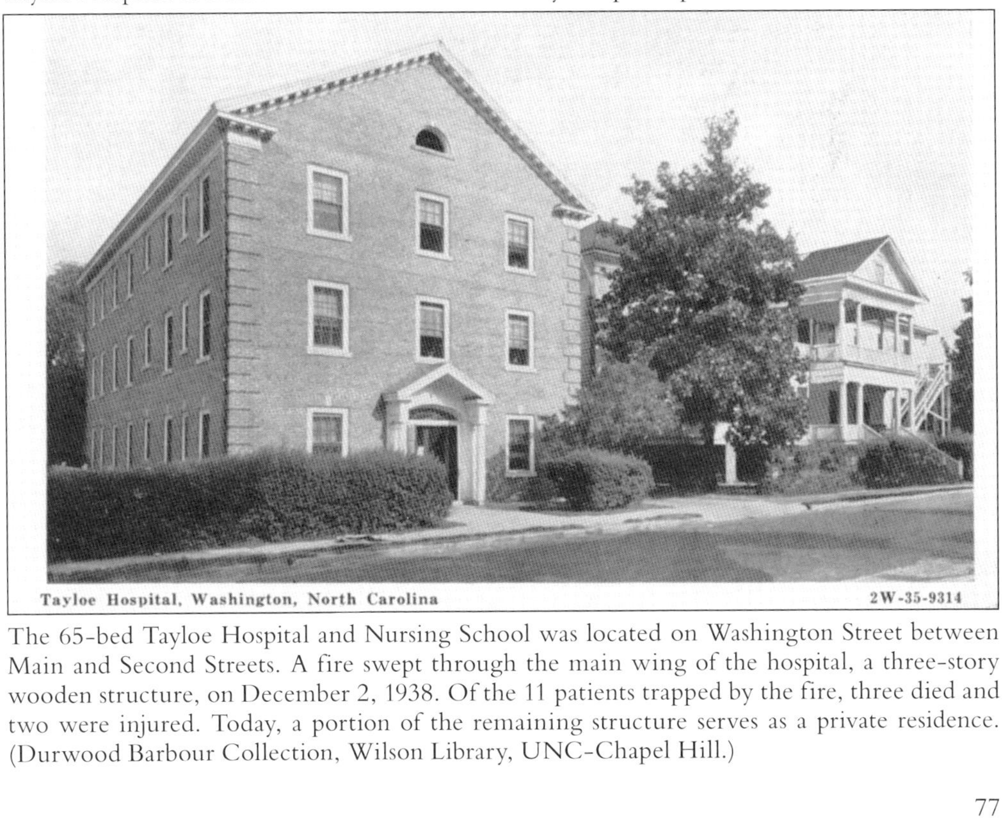
Tayloe Hospital, Washington, North Carolina
2W-35-9314

The 65-bed Tayloe Hospital and Nursing School was located on Washington Street between Main and Second Streets. A fire swept through the main wing of the hospital, a three-story wooden structure, on December 2, 1938. Of the 11 patients trapped by the fire, three died and two were injured. Today, a portion of the remaining structure serves as a private residence. (Durwood Barbour Collection, Wilson Library, UNC-Chapel Hill.)

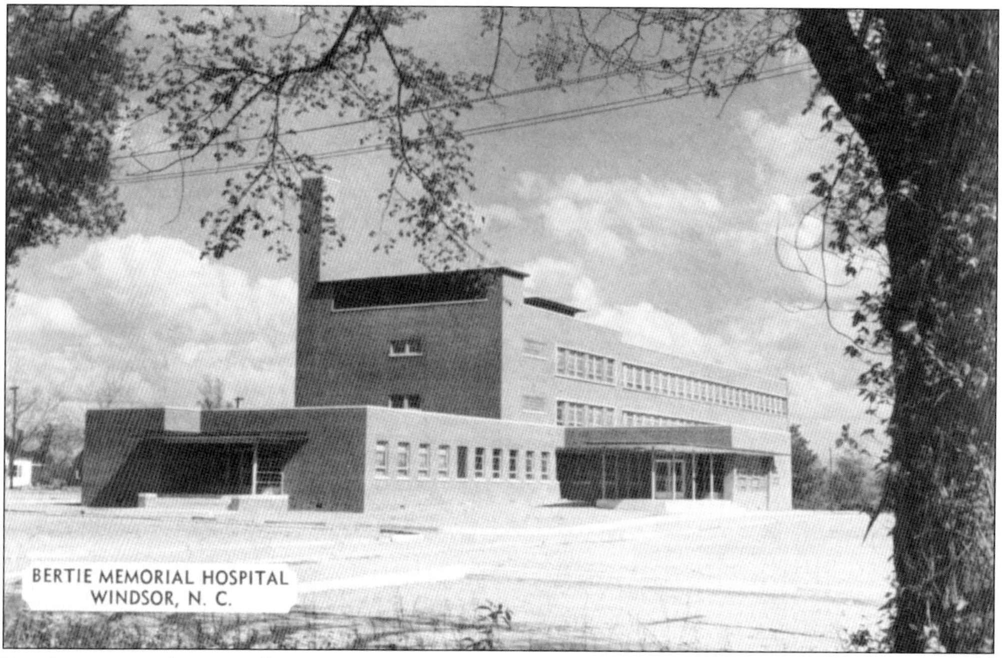

Bertie Memorial Hospital, supported by Hill-Burton funds, opened in 1952 in Windsor (Bertie County). It briefly closed in 1985. The organization known today as Vidant Health took over operations in 1998 and built a replacement structure based on Critical Access Hospital (CAH) standards. The original hospital, located at 401 Sterlingworth Street, is now an apartment building. (Durwood Barbour Collection, Wilson Library, UNC-Chapel Hill.)

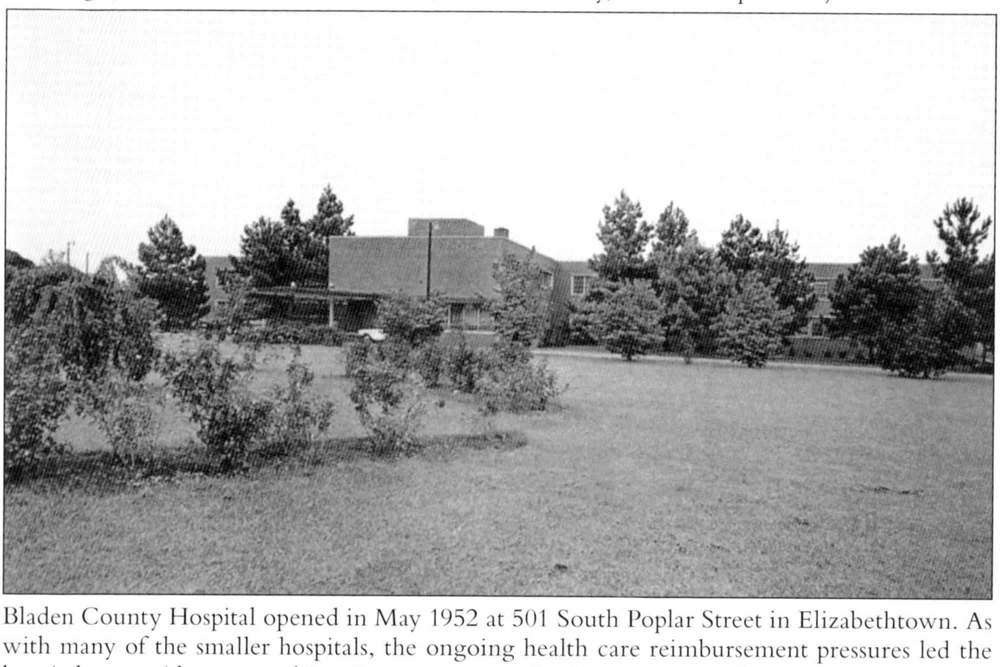

Bladen County Hospital opened in May 1952 at 501 South Poplar Street in Elizabethtown. As with many of the smaller hospitals, the ongoing health care reimbursement pressures led the hospital to consider partnerships. A request to area health care systems led to a 2008 agreement with Cape Fear Valley Health System in nearby Fayetteville. Today, it is the Cape Fear Valley Bladen County Hospital, operated as a CAH.

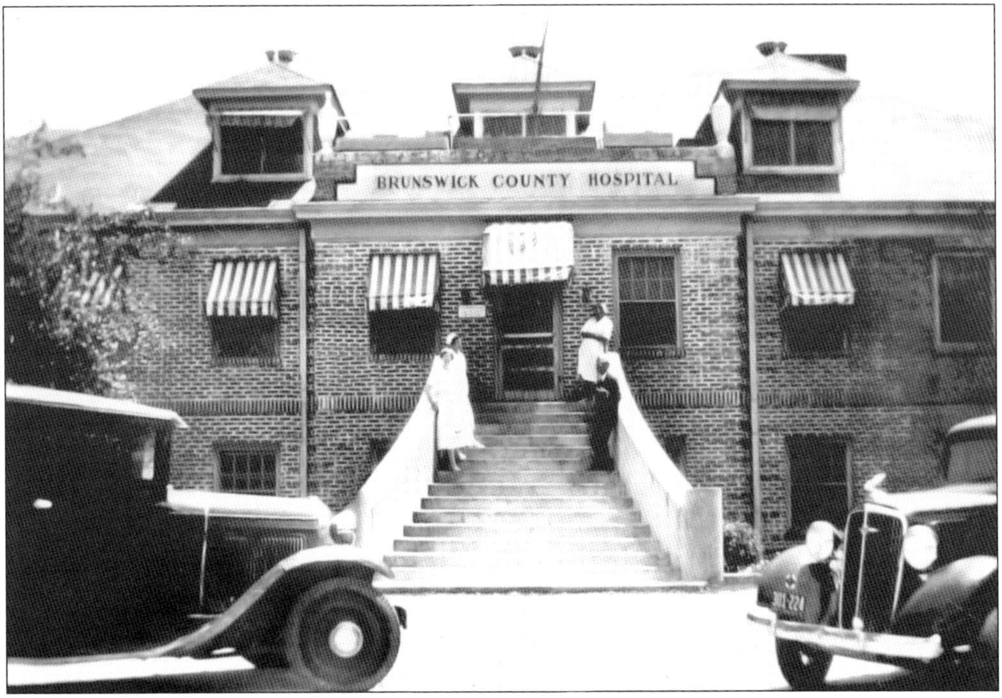

The Brunswick County Hospital opened on June 2, 1930, at 924 North Howe Street in Southport. An area surgeon, Dr. Julius Arthur Dosher, the acting assistant surgeon in the US Public Health Service, was stationed at the Southport Quarantine Station. He also saw patients at the Brunswick County Hospital. Shortly after his death of TB complications, the hospital was renamed the J. Arthur Dosher Memorial Hospital. (*State Port Pilot* newspaper).

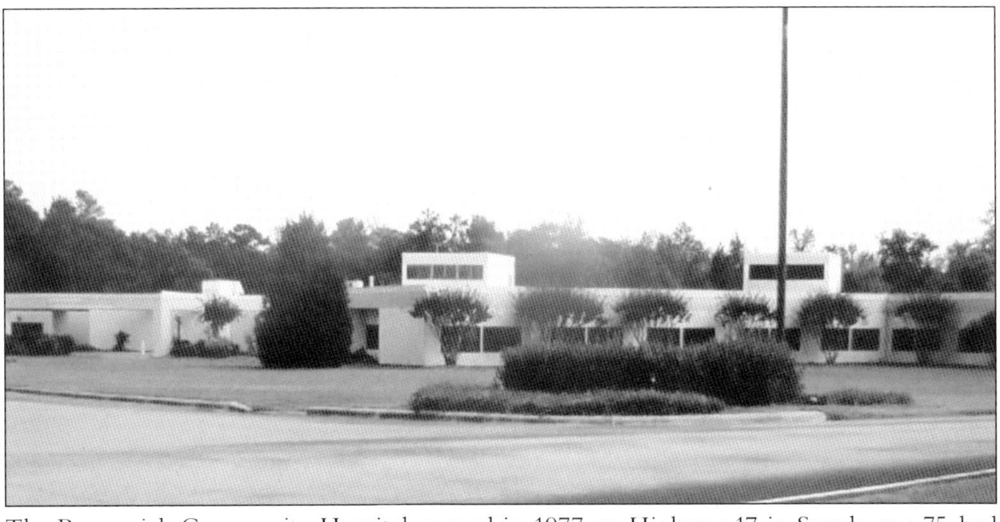

The Brunswick Community Hospital opened in 1977 on Highway 17 in Supply as a 75-bed hospital. For a time, the hospital was operated as Brunswick Columbia/HCA, in the Columbia/HCA network. In 2006, the hospital merged with the Novant Health System, becoming the Brunswick Novant Medical Center. In 2011, a 74-bed replacement hospital opened just north of the old hospital campus in Bolivia. (North Carolina State Archives.)

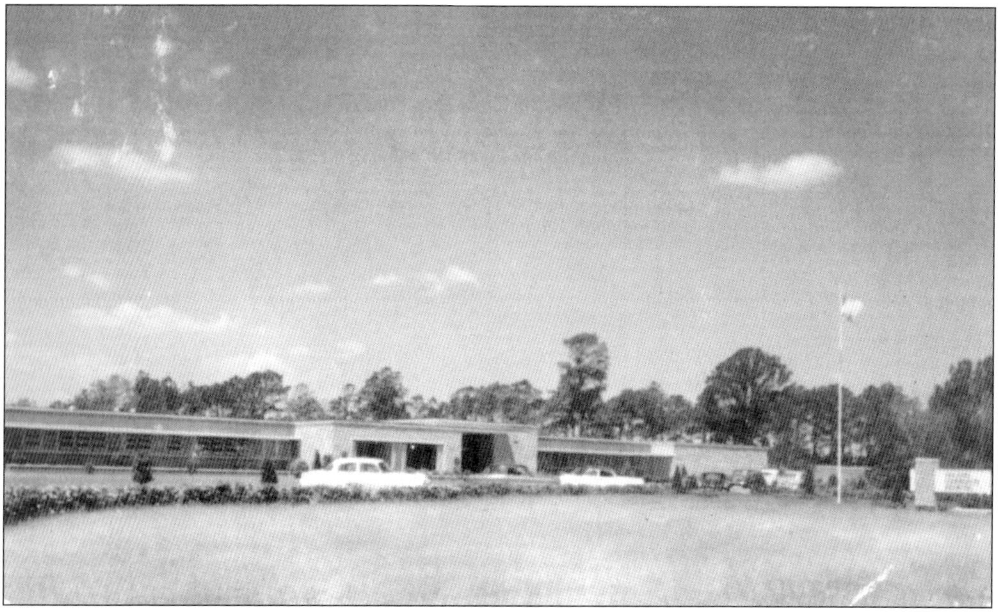

The Sea Level (Sealevel) and Atlantic communities (Carteret County), at the terminus of Highway 70, relying in part on Hill-Burton funding, opened a small general hospital in 1953. The Sea Level Hospital was "given" to the Duke University Medical System in 1969. Several efforts to keep the hospital open included Carteret General using the facility for rehabilitation, but by 2005, it was sold and converted to a skilled nursing facility.

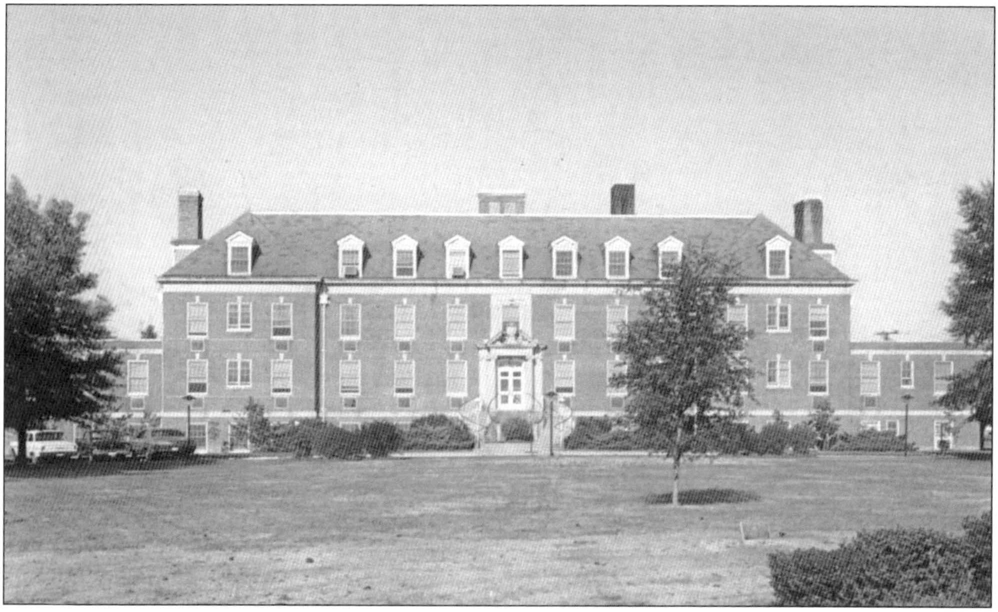

The Roanoke-Chowan Hospital opened in 1948 in Ahoskie (Hertford County) at the corner of South Academy Street and Memorial Drive. It was the first American hospital to use the Hill-Burton funding for hospital construction. By 1959, it was a 107-bed hospital. A replacement facility was built on-site in 1970. In 1996, it joined the University Health System of Eastern Carolina (Vidant Health) and is now known as Vidant Roanoke-Chowan Hospital. (Durwood Barbour Collection, Wilson Library, UNC-Chapel Hill.)

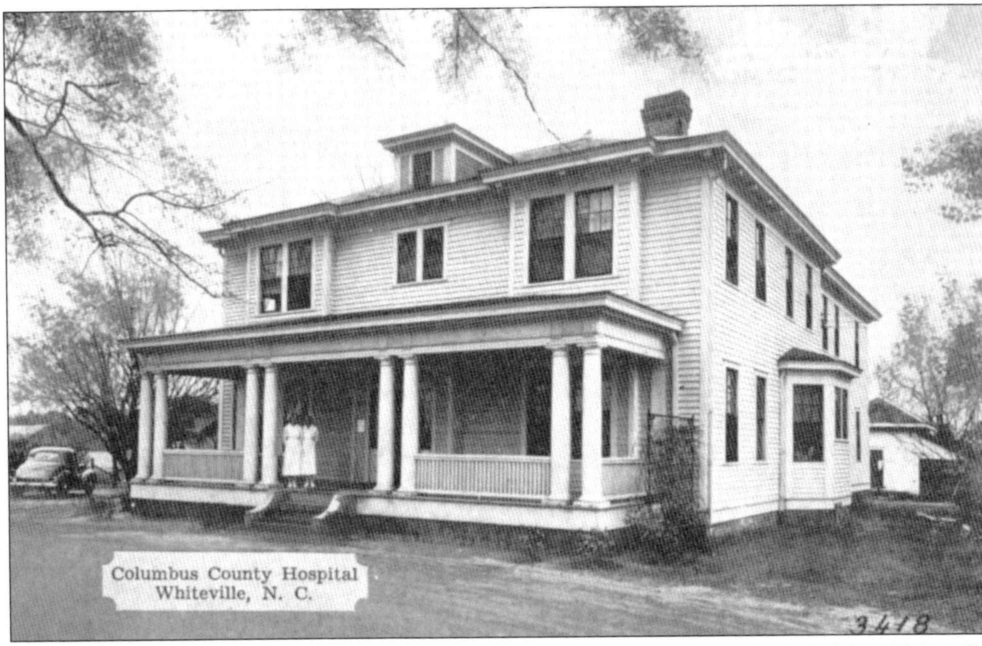

Dr. Warren Edward Miller established the 12-bed Columbus County Hospital in Whiteville in 1935. A 60-bed hospital opened in March 1940. The current Jefferson Street facility opened in 1977. Today, the 154-bed Columbus Regional Health Care System is managed by Carolinas Health Care System. (Durwood Barbour Collection, Wilson Library, UNC-Chapel Hill.)

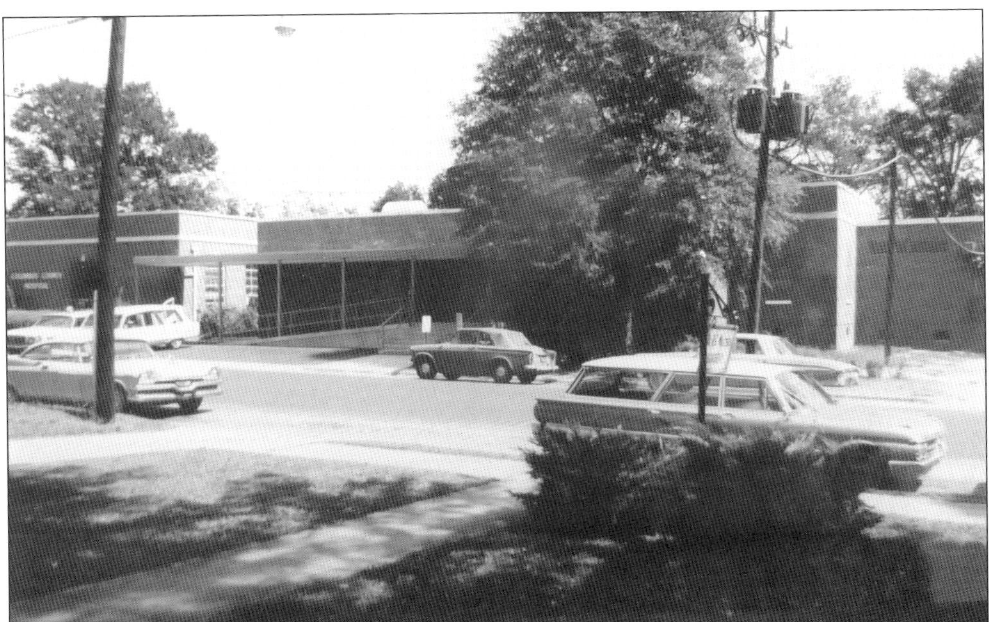
The Columbus County Hospital completed a 46-bed addition (pictured here) in 1965 to include outpatient services and expand the emergency department. (North Carolina State Archives.)

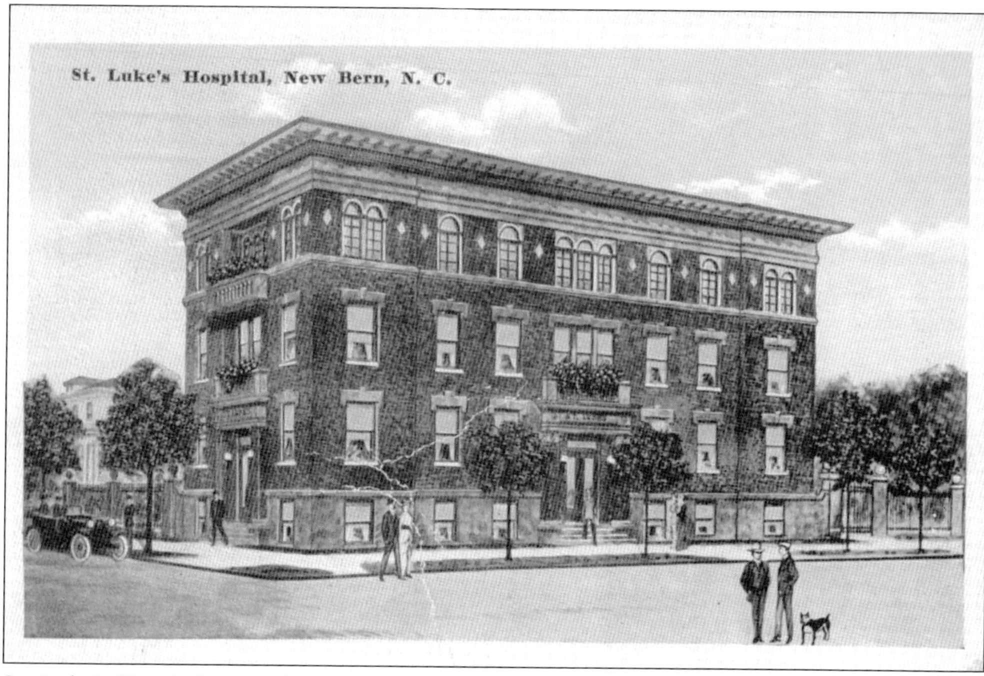

St. Luke's Hospital opened in 1914 at 403 Broad Street, at the corner of George Street, in New Bern. The Sisters of St. Josephs, of Newark, New Jersey, purchased St. Luke's in 1944. A three-story addition on the George Street side more than doubled the facility to 65 beds and 20 bassinets. It was seldom financially stable. In 1961, local citizens approved funding to build a consolidated Craven County Hospital.

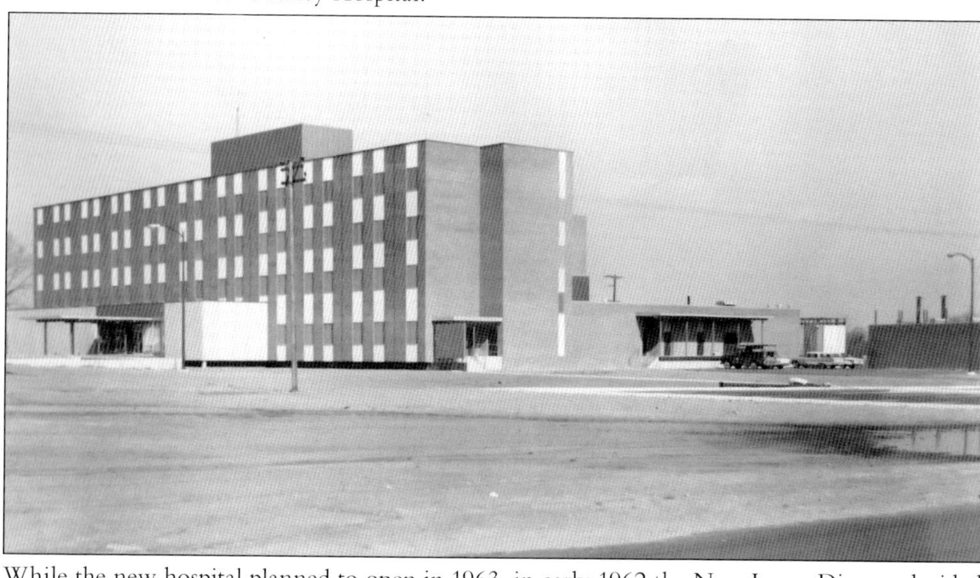

While the new hospital planned to open in 1963, in early 1962 the New Jersey Diocese decided to immediately close St. Luke's based on financial peril. Local leaders quickly negotiated a purchase. The St. Luke's building became the temporary Craven County Hospital. The 100-bed Craven County Hospital opened in 1963. Today, known as the CarolinaEast Health System, the 350-bed hospital anchors a comprehensive health care system for the region. (North Carolina State Archives.)

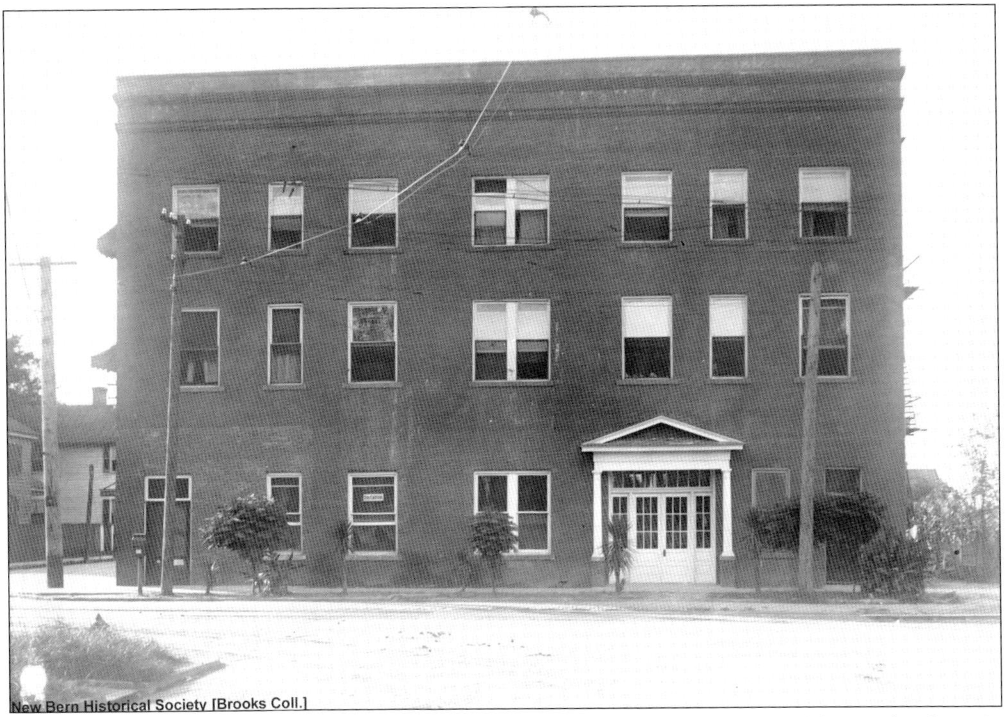

In 1912, the Fairview Hospital Corporation opened a 20-bed private general hospital. This 22-bed hospital was operated by Dr. George A. Caton and routinely referred to as Canton Hospital. After Dr. Caton's death, the hospital closed, and the structure was used as an apartment building until being purchased by the Salvation Army. At the time, the name of the street was Griffith Street, now known as North Craven Street, at the corner of Queen Street. (New Bern Historical Society, Brooks Collection.)

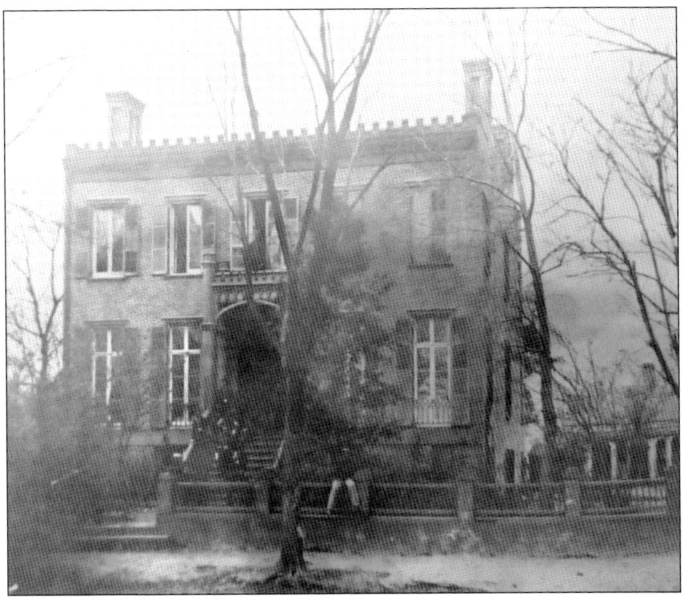

Kafer Memorial Hospital opened in 1949 as a nonprofit 42-bed, nine-bassinet general hospital by Dr. Oscar Kafer, a local surgeon. It occupied the former Hughes home at 509 Broad Street. It was acquired by the Atlantic Baptist Association on January 3, 1958. The thought that the North Carolina Baptist Hospital in Winston Salem would join the effort to help operate the hospital never materialized. The hospital closed in November 1959. (UNC Southern Historical Collection.)

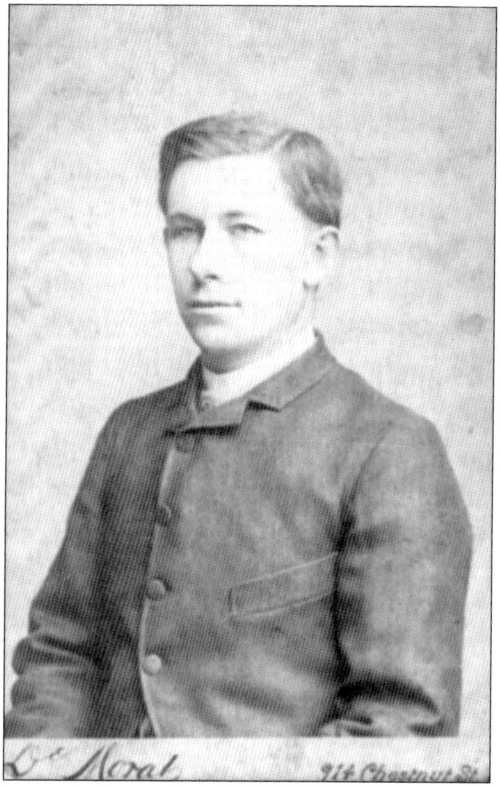

Jacob Franklin Highsmith opened a doctor's office in Fayetteville on Green Street, with rooms above for patients who needed to stay overnight, in 1896. In 1899, Dr. J.H. Marsh joined Dr. Highsmith, and the facility expanded to Market Street. It became known as the Marsh-Highsmith Sanatorium. In 1902, Dr. Highsmith purchased Dr. Marsh's interest, and it was renamed Highsmith Hospital. (Archive.org.)

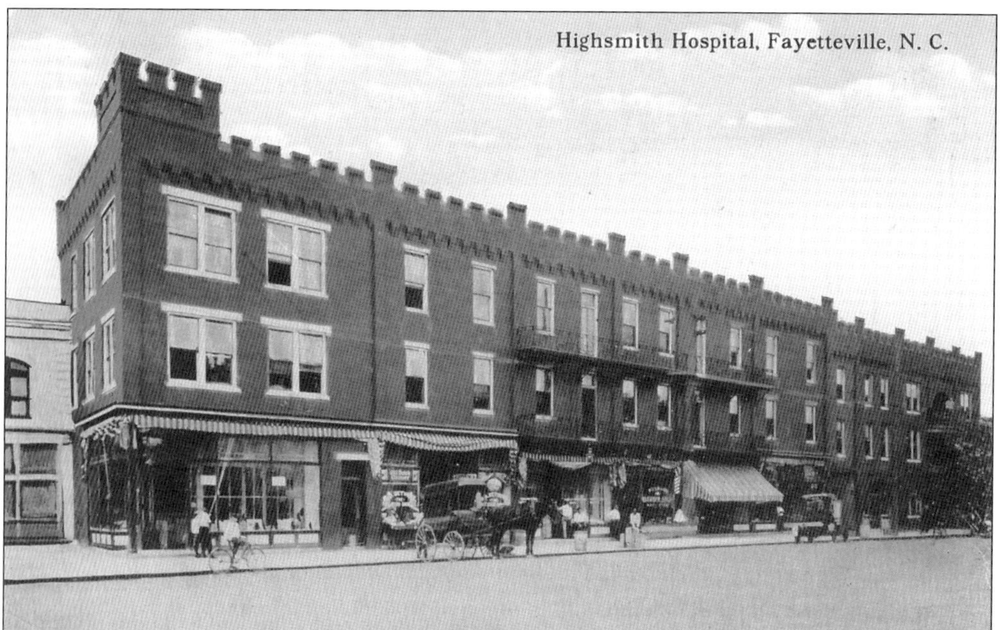

In 1913, Dr. W.T. Rainey joined Highsmith Hospital, and it continued to thrive, known at the time as one of the most modern and aptly equipped in the state. By 1923, the 75-bed hospital included operating rooms, a nurse training program, and an ambulance, and it was one of the first hospitals in the state approved to use insulin for diabetic patients.

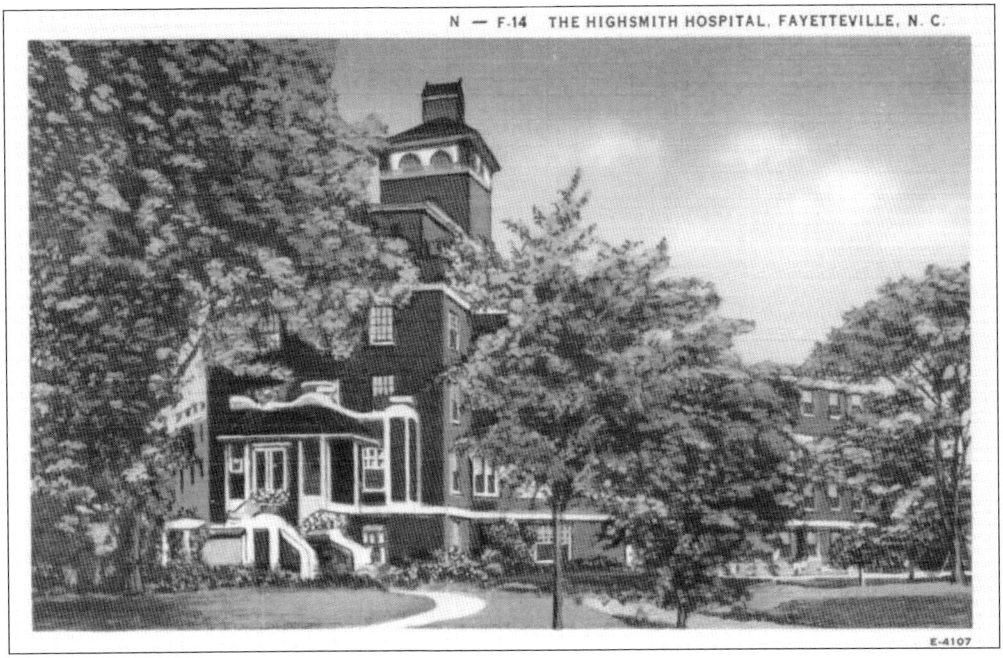

Highsmith Hospital was limited in growth due to its location, and as such, a new hospital was opened in 1926 in Fayetteville. The hospital later became known as the Highsmith-Rainey Hospital. In the 1990s, the hospital was purchased by Columbia-Hospital Corporation of America (more commonly known as Columbia/HCA). In 2000, the hospital was acquired by the Cape Fear Valley Health System.

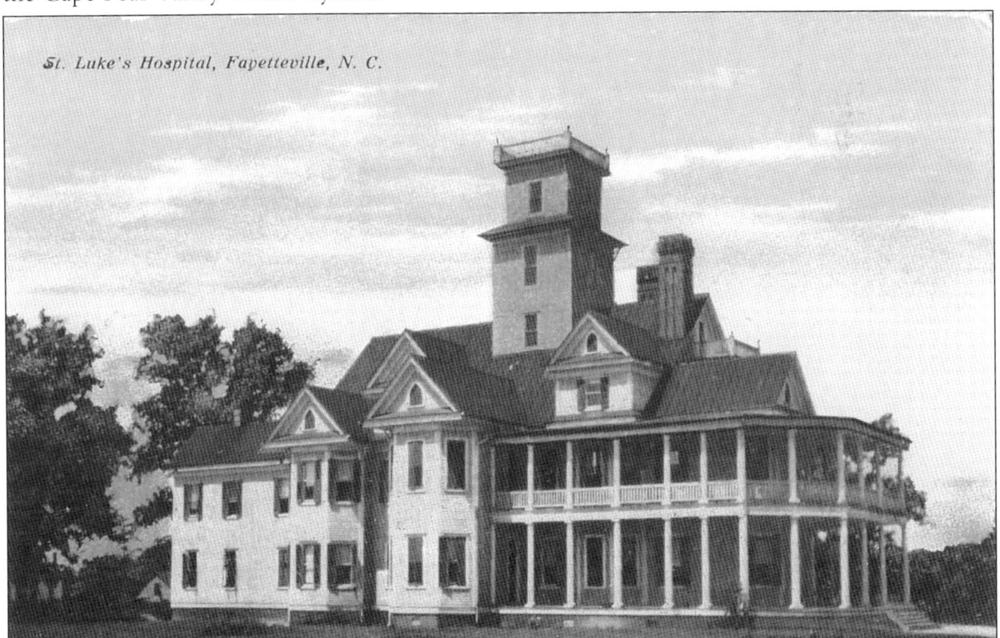

In 1905, the St. Luke's Hospital opened in Fayetteville as St. Luke's Sanatorium. In 1914, it was a 32-bed hospital with doctors R.B. Hayes and T.M. West as the PICs. By 1916, the hospital was no longer listed in the AMA Hospital Registry.

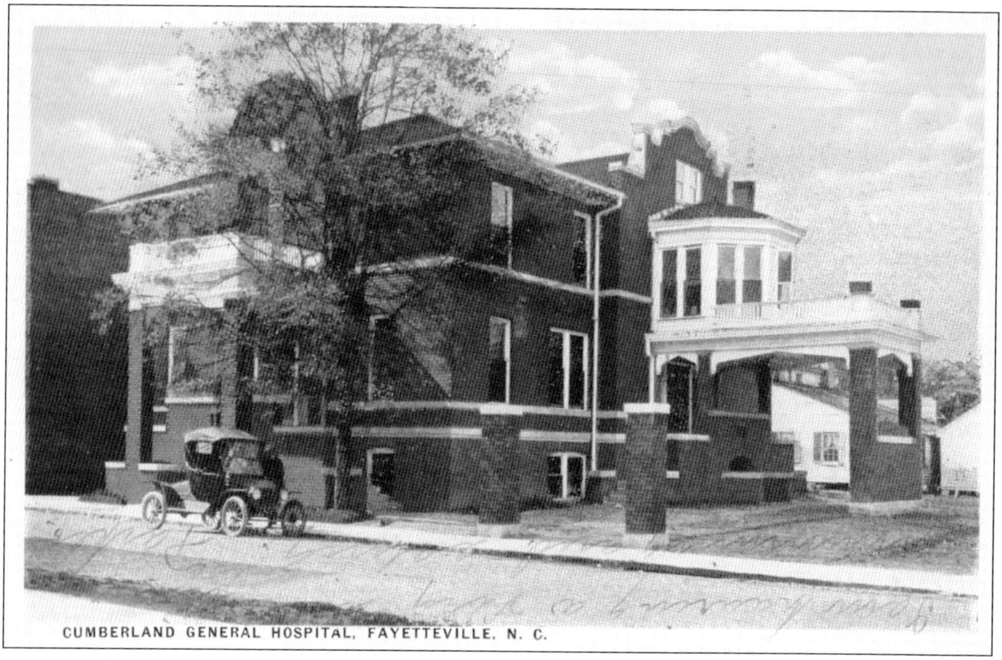

In 1913, the Fayetteville Infirmary, also known as Cumberland General Hospital, opened at 218 Old Lumberton Road. In 1923, the 30-bed hospital included doctors T.M. West and Seavy Highsmith serving as the PICs. A 1923 advertisement touted the Fayetteville hospital for "The Treatment of Medical and Surgical Diseases" with a "School for Nurses, Three Year Course."

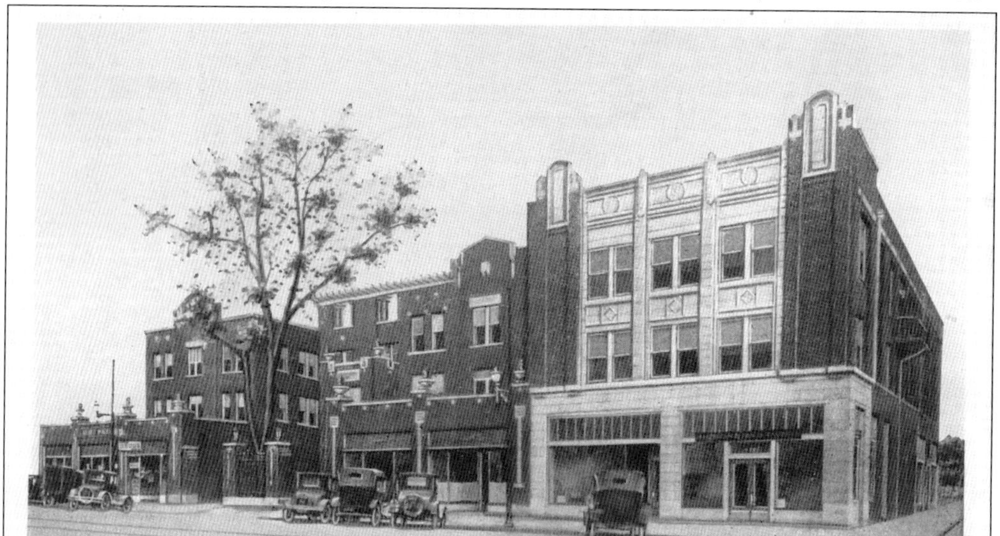

In 1919, the 56-bed Pittman Hospital was opened in Fayetteville by Dr. R.L. Pittman. Dr. Pittman was an exceptional surgeon. However, the hospital later achieved unfavorable notoriety; *Pate v. RL Pittman Hospital Inc. et al.* (1951) dealt with a patient being held in the hospital after being cleared for discharge because "she failed to pay her hospital bill." With Dr. Pittman's failing health, the hospital closed in 1954.

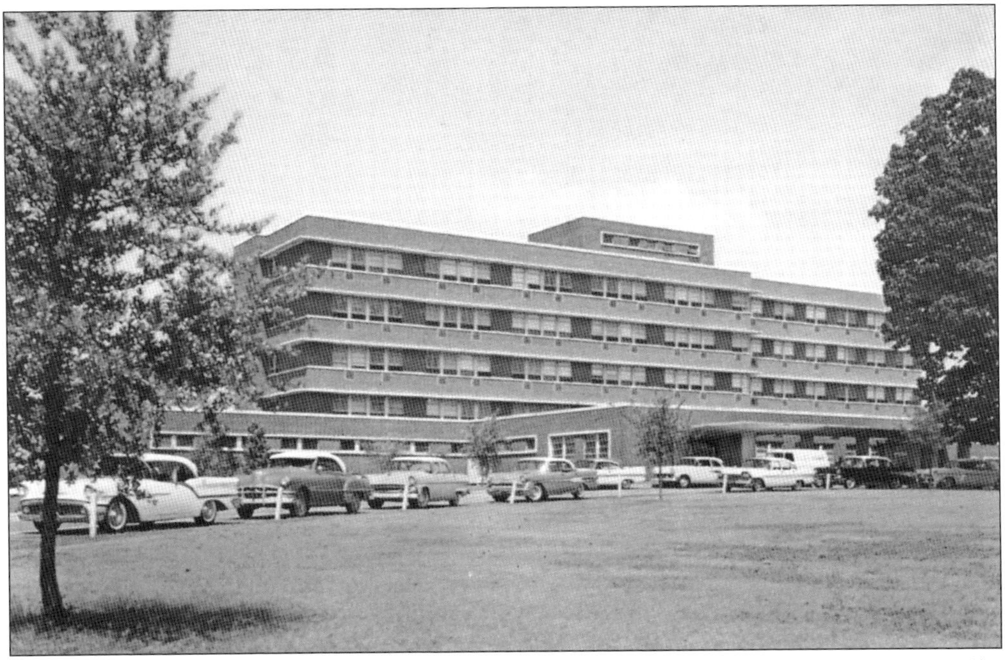

In 1956, the 200-bed Cumberland County Hospital opened at 1638 Owen Drive in Fayetteville. Today, the 592-bed hospital is known as the Cape Fear Valley Medical Center and anchors the Cape Fear Valley Health System.

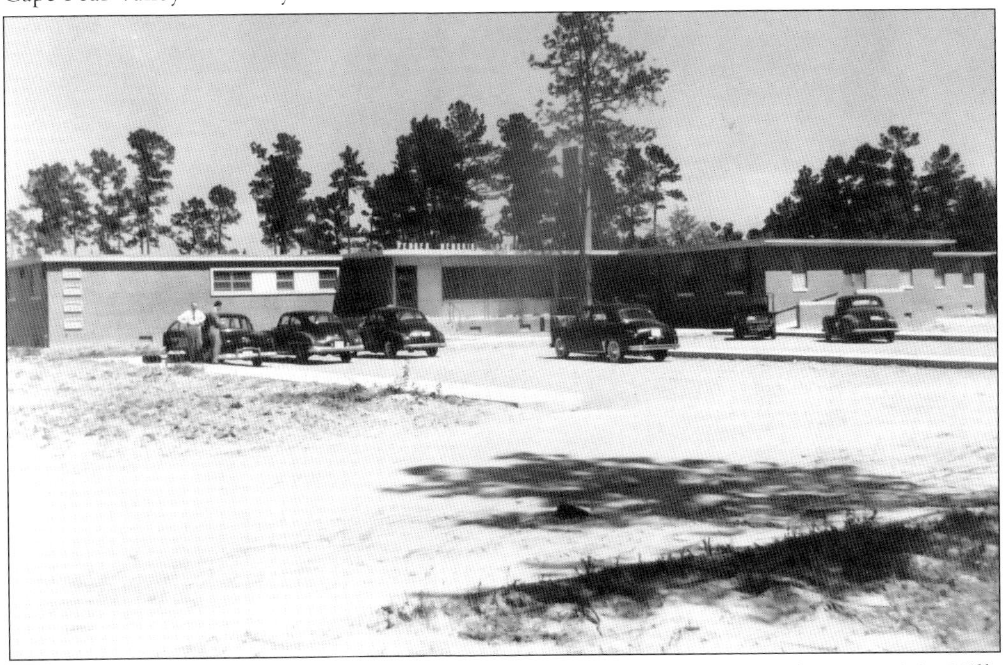

On May 18, 1951, relying on a $50,000 bond approved by the voters and $200,000 in Hill-Burton funding, the 25-bed Pender Memorial Hospital opened in Burgaw. Although once a 45-bed hospital with a 43-bed skilled nursing facility, today it is operated as a 25-bed CAH. The county-owned hospital is managed by the New Hanover Regional Health Care System. (North Carolina State Archives.)

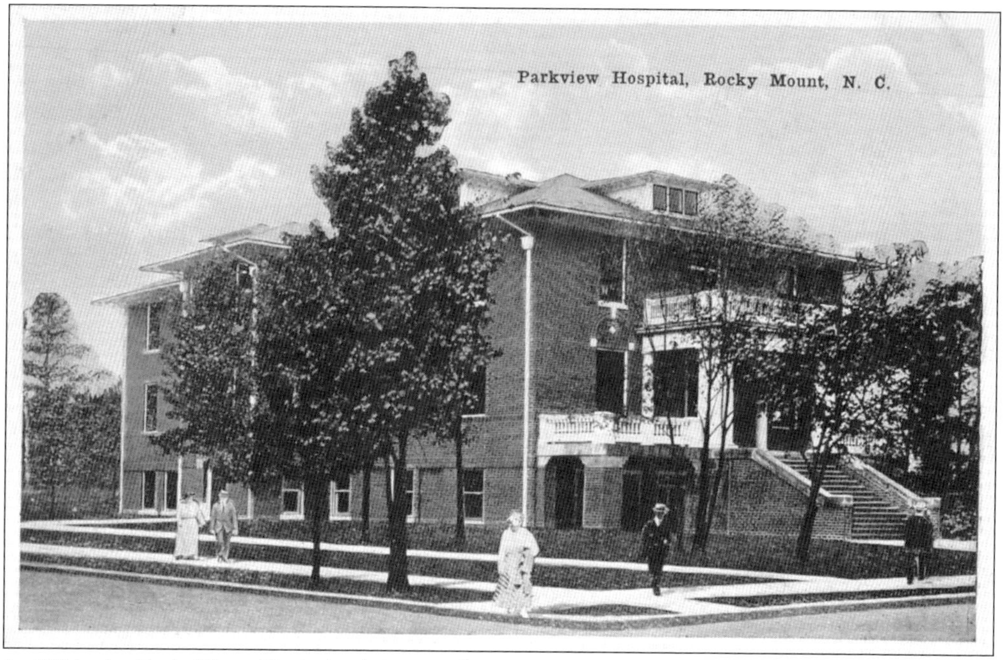

In 1914, the Park View (Parkview) Hospital opened at the corner of Falls Road and Hickory Street in Rocky Mount (Edgecombe/Nash Counties). Doctors J.P. Whitehead, I.P. Battle, E.B. Quillen, R.H. Speight, J.P. Speight, George B. Johnston, and Dr. A. Murat Willis opened the hospital. A surgeon from Richmond joined them shortly thereafter, Dr. Edmund S. Boyce, who, along with Dr. Willis, purchased the hospital from the group the following year.

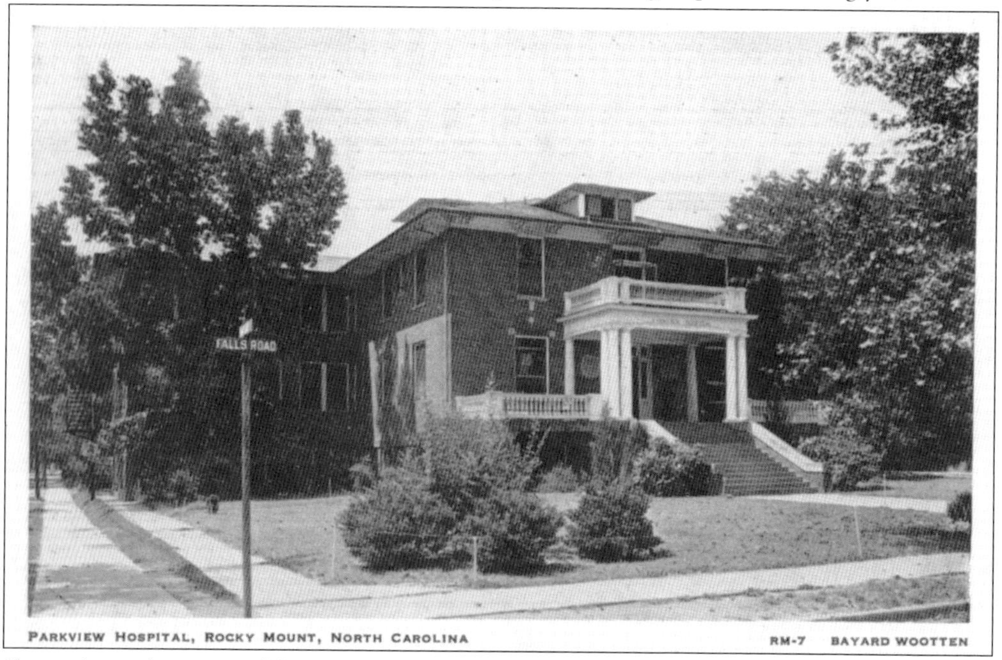

Shown is another view of the Parkview Hospital with the expansion wing that added additional beds on the west side of the hospital. By 1923, Dr. Edmund Boyce and Dr. A. Murat Willis were the PICs for the 70-bed hospital.

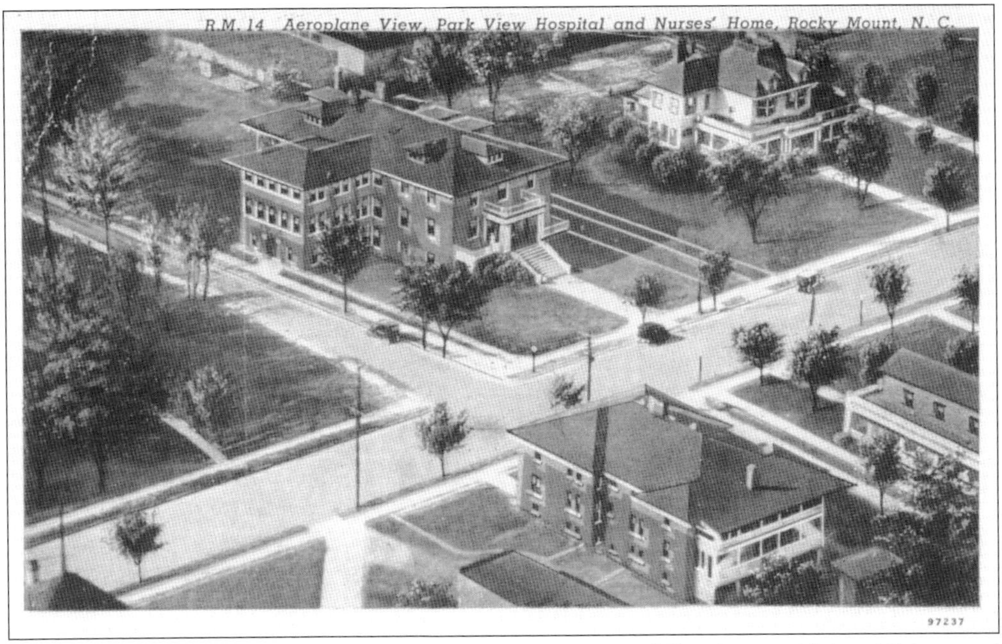
R.M. 14 Aeroplane View, Park View Hospital and Nurses' Home, Rocky Mount, N. C.
97237

Shown here is the Park View Hospital and Nurses Home following multiple additions and renovations. Park View added air-conditioning in 1954 and was a state-of-the-art facility at the time. The Rocky Mount area hospitals were replaced in 1971 by Nash General Hospital. Nash UNC Health Care is today a 292-bed facility.

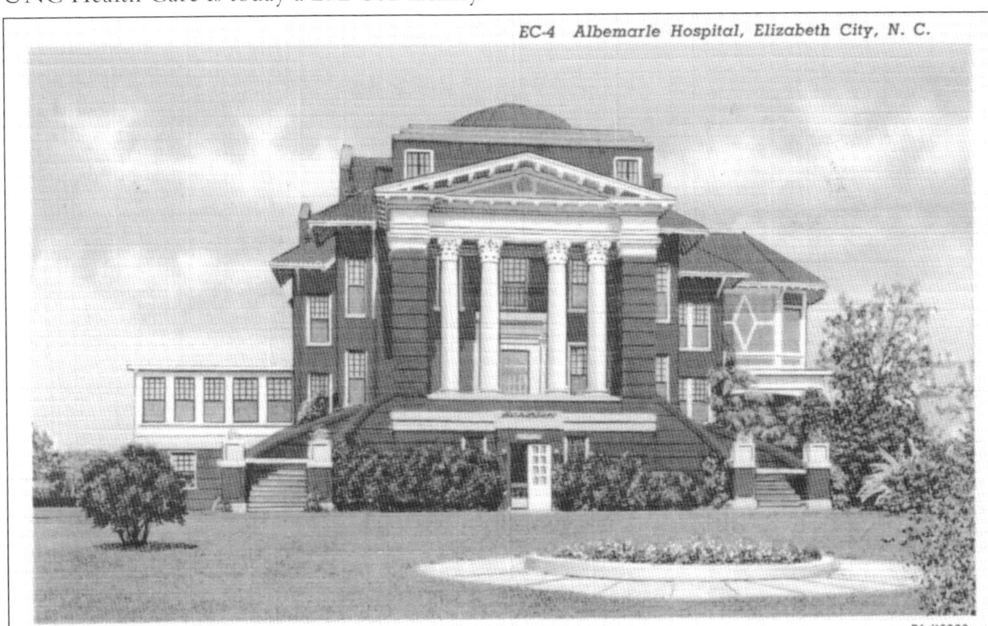
EC-4 Albemarle Hospital, Elizabeth City, N. C.
7A-H2999

In 1914, the original Albemarle Hospital opened on Riverside Avenue in Elizabeth City. In 1923, the 45-bed hospital was identified as Pasquotank Municipal Hospital Association, Inc. Elizabeth City is located on the Albemarle Sound, next to the intercoastal waterway that connects much of the East Coast. The city is a common harbor for pleasure boats, shipping, and commerce.

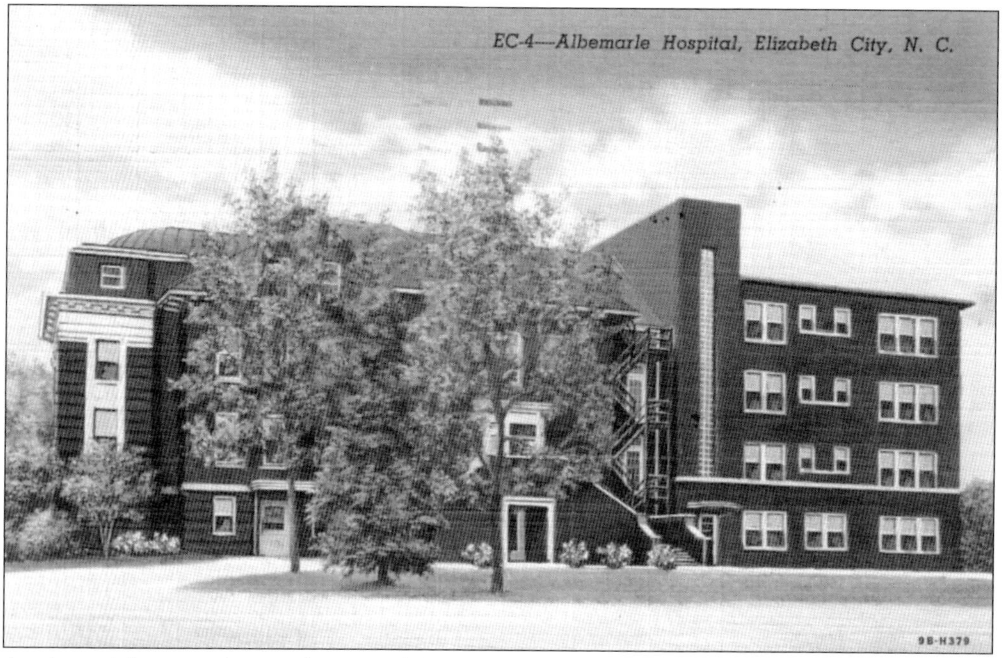

A substantial renovation to the rear of the Albemarle Hospital almost doubled the size in the 1950s. Pictured above is the original facility facing left and the new addition at right.

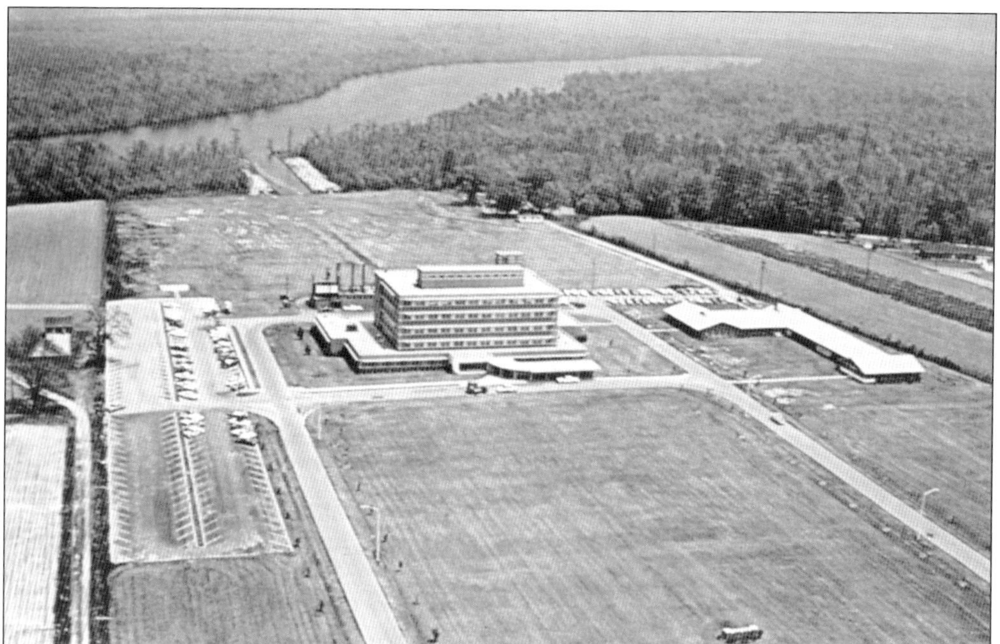
In 1960, the Albemarle Hospital built a 200-bed replacement facility to better serve the region. In 2009, the hospital aligned with Vidant Health (in Greenville). By 2013, the Vidant relationship had soured, and the Pasquotank County Commissioners accepted a long-term lease (40 years) of the hospital with Sentara Health (a Norfolk, Virginia–based hospital system). Today, the hospital is known as Sentara Albemarle Hospital.

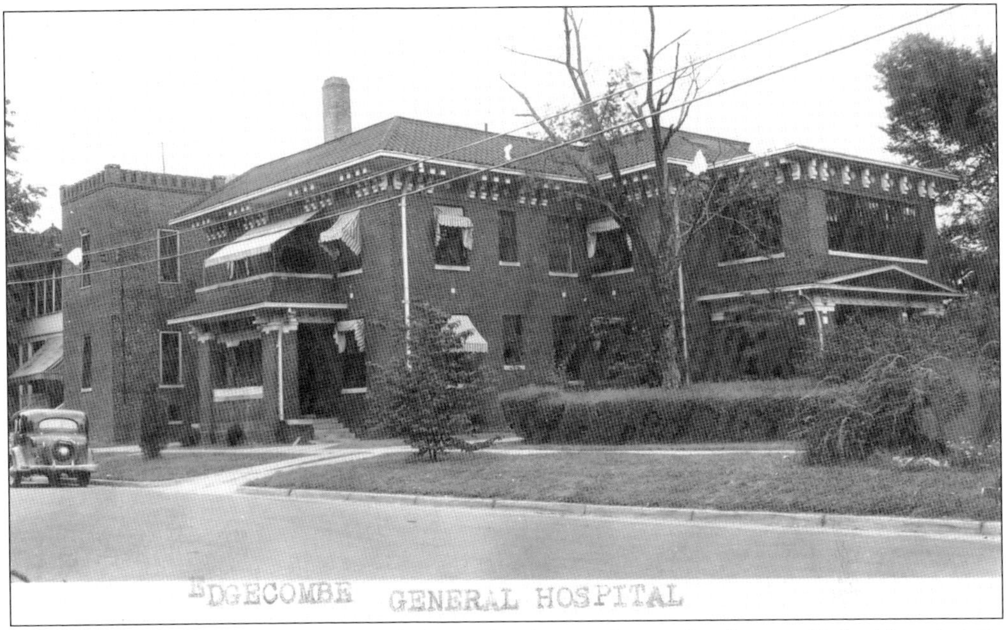

In 1916, Edgecombe County General (formerly Pittman Sanatorium) was a 60-bed hospital. In 1959, relying on Hill-Burton funds, Edgecombe County hospitals merged into a new building on North Main Street, in Tarboro. Hospital Corporation of America purchased the facility in 1982 and built a replacement named Heritage Hospital. In 1998, it was purchased by Vidant and is now Vidant Edgecombe Hospital. (Digital NC, Edgecombe County Memorial Library.)

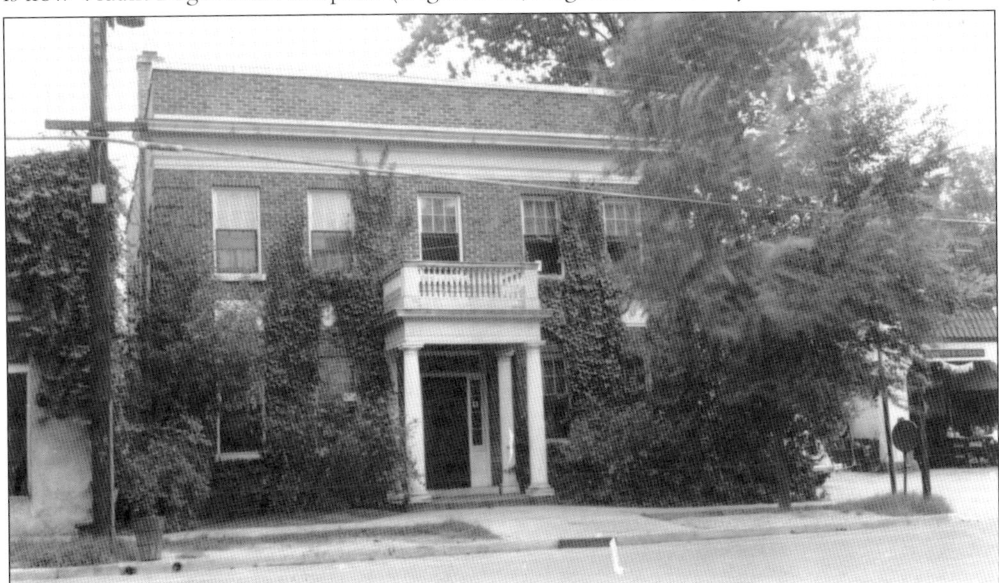

In 1929, the eight-bed Bass Memorial Hospital was opened in Tarboro at 119 West James Street by Dr. Spencer P. Bass. The hospital was named in honor of his father, Dr. Henry Turner Bass, who died of a gunshot wound in 1903. Dr. Bass specialized in pediatric care. The hospital closed in 1959 when it merged with the other Edgecombe County hospitals. (Digital NC, Edgecombe County Memorial Library.)

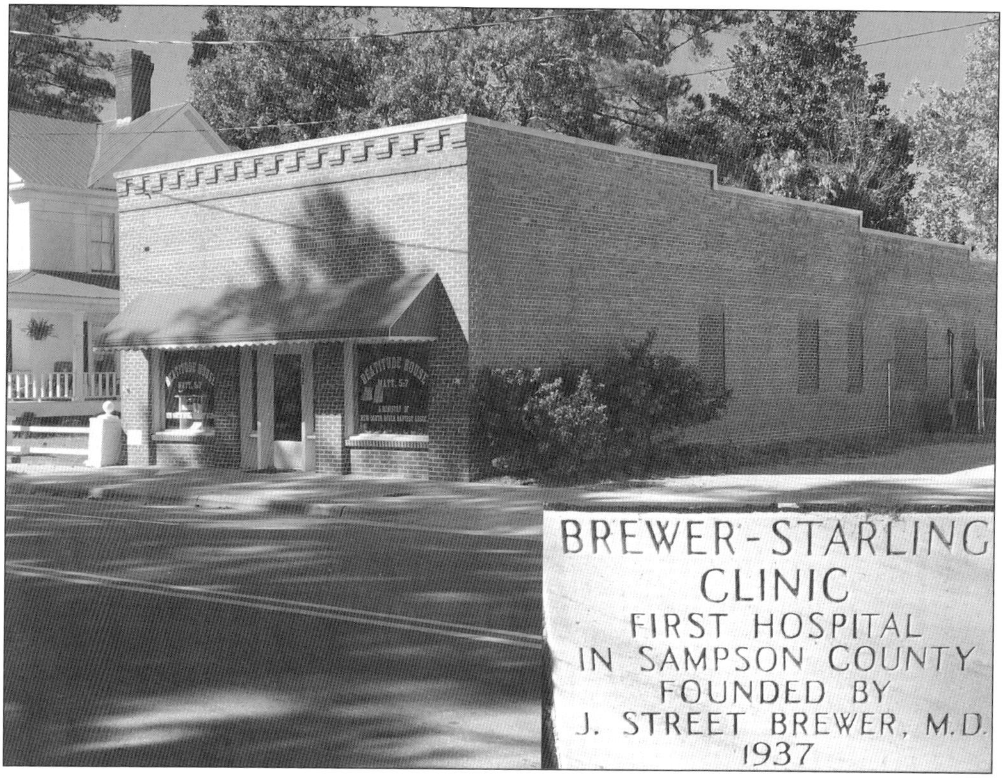
BREWER-STARLING
CLINIC
FIRST HOSPITAL
IN SAMPSON COUNTY
FOUNDED BY
J. STREET BREWER, M.D.
1937

Dr. James S. Brewer grew up in Roseboro as his father was the local school superintendent. After attending Wake Forest College, he returned to Roseboro in 1920 and began practicing medicine. He was joined by Dr. Plato Starling, and in 1937, they established the Brewer Starling Clinic (Hospital) at 212 West Roseboro Street. This nine-bed, five-bassinet facility was the first hospital serving Sampson County. It operated as a hospital until the early 1960s, when Sampson Memorial Hospital replaced the hospital services for the county. Dr. Starling died in 1968. The clinic closed with Dr. Brewer's retirement in 1974.

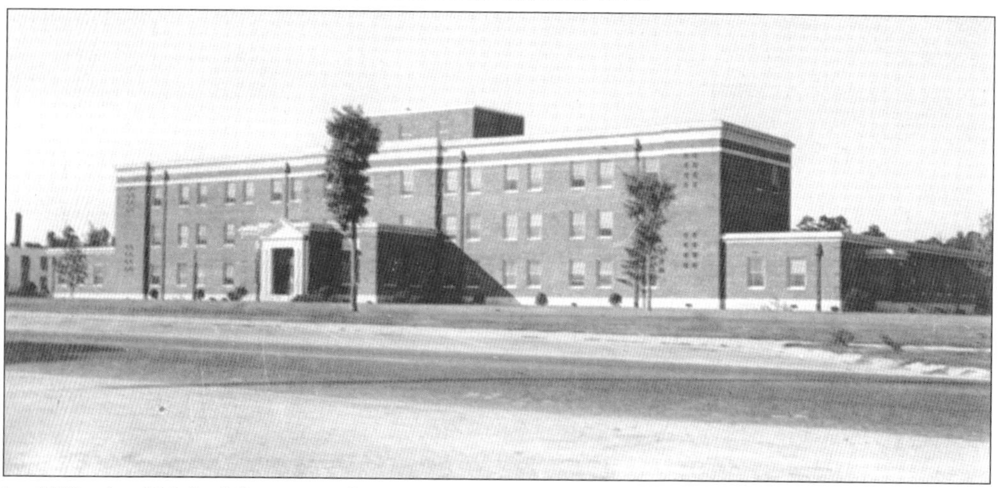

In 1950, the 100-bed Sampson County Memorial Hospital opened at 607 Beaman Street in Clinton. The Sampson Regional Medical Center today is a 146-bed facility. (Durwood Barbour Collection, Wilson Library, UNC-Chapel Hill.)

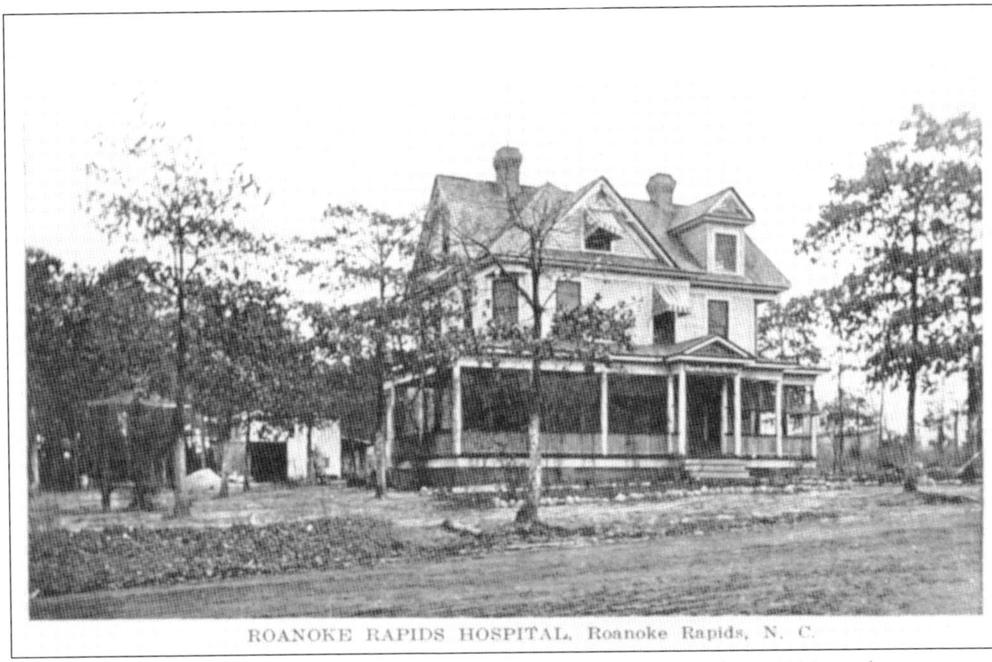

In 1914, the Roanoke Rapids Hospital (Halifax County) opened in 1914 at the corner of Roanoke Avenue and Seventh Street (where Veterans Park is located today). In 1923, the 50-bed hospital listed Dr. W.M. Long as the PIC. Relying in part on Hill-Burton funding, a new and much larger replacement hospital was built in 1972. (Durwood Barbour Collection, Wilson Library, UNC-Chapel Hill.)

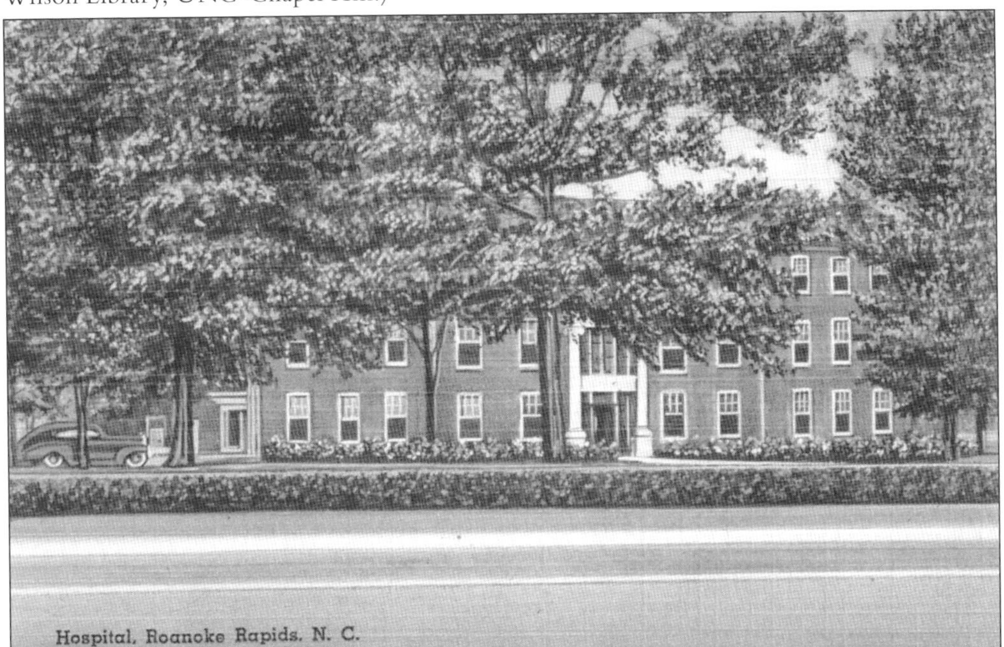

Opened in 1972 at 250 Smith Church Road, the 150-bed Halifax County Hospital replaced the Roanoke Avenue facility. Today, Halifax Regional Medical Center is a 204-bed hospital serving the patients of a six-county region.

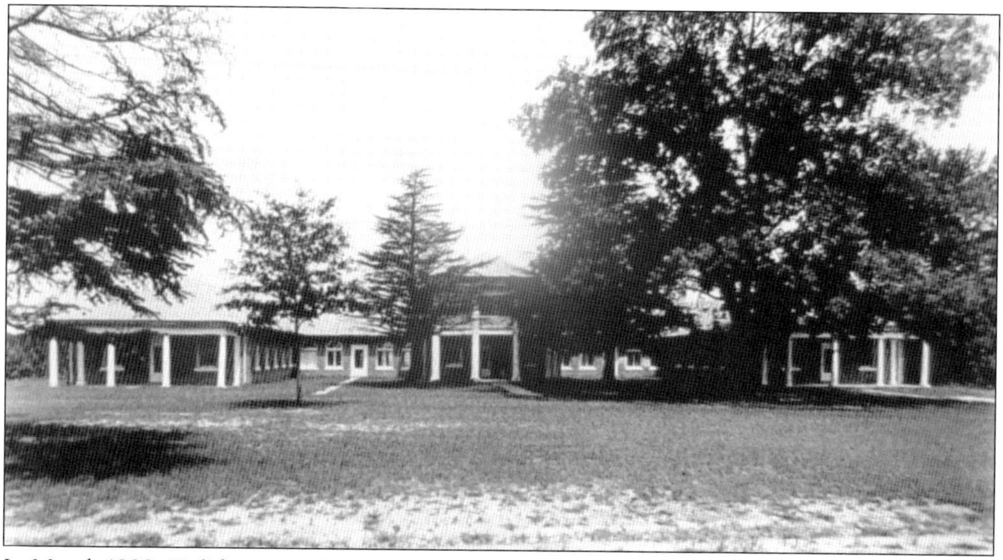

In March 1922, Halifax commissioners approved the construction of the Halifax County Home and Tubercular Hospital to improve health care for the indigent during the early 20th century. The building was constructed on NC 903 near State Route 1667. The home transitioned to a county rest home in 1959 before being abandoned in 1972. Today, this restored county building is in the National Register of Historic Places. (North Carolina State Archives.)

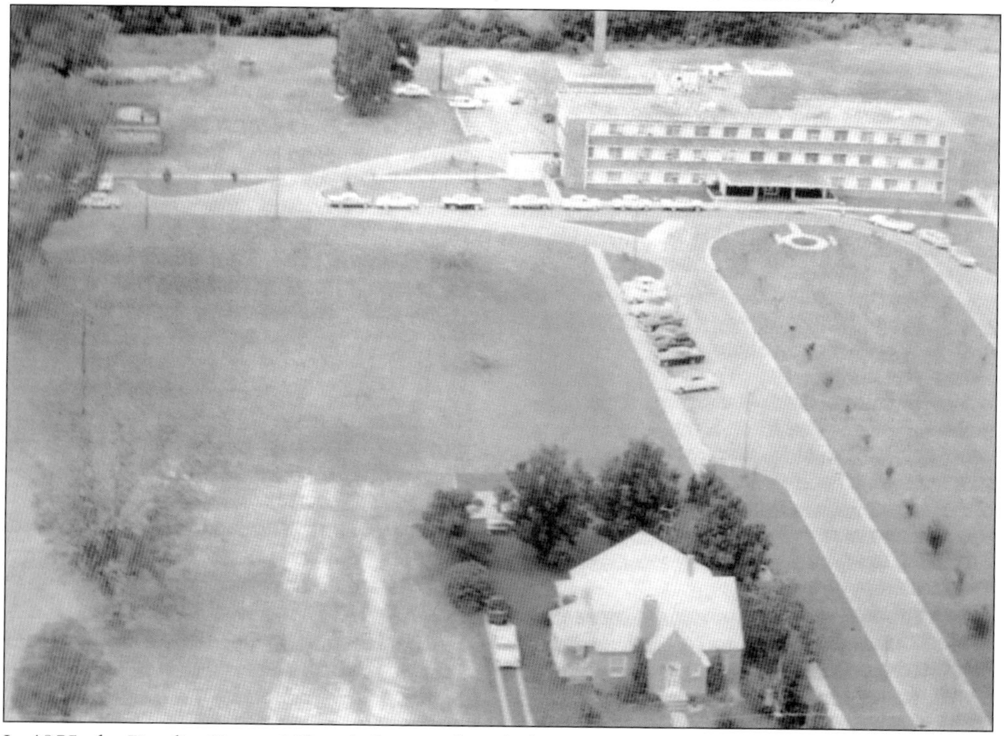

In 1955, the Duplin General Hospital opened with the aid of Hill-Burton funding in Kenansville at 401 North Main Street. Over the years, the hospital added skilled nursing and behavioral health beds, taking it to a 101-bed hospital. It has since partnered with the Vidant Health, and today the Vidant Duplin Hospital is operated as a CAH. (North Carolina State Archives.)

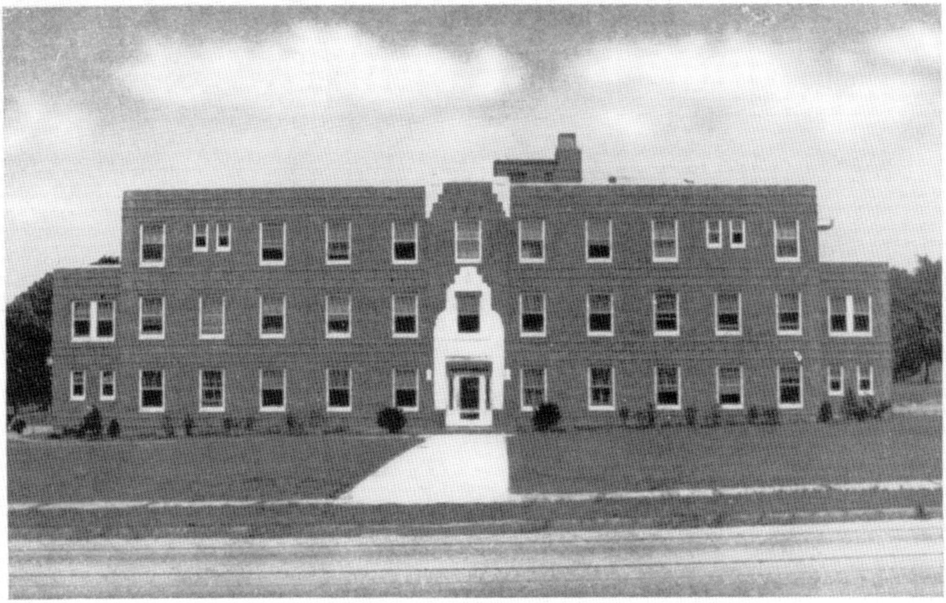

Harnett County Hospital ($110,000 Building), Dunn, North Carolina

Originally opened as Dunn Hospital on North Ellis Street, the hospital was renamed Betsy Johnson Hospital in 1956. The 101-bed hospital moved to its current Tilghman Drive location in 1968. A second Harnett Health hospital was built in Lillington in 2005, known as Central Harnett Hospital. Both Harnett hospitals are operated by the Cape Fear Valley Health System.

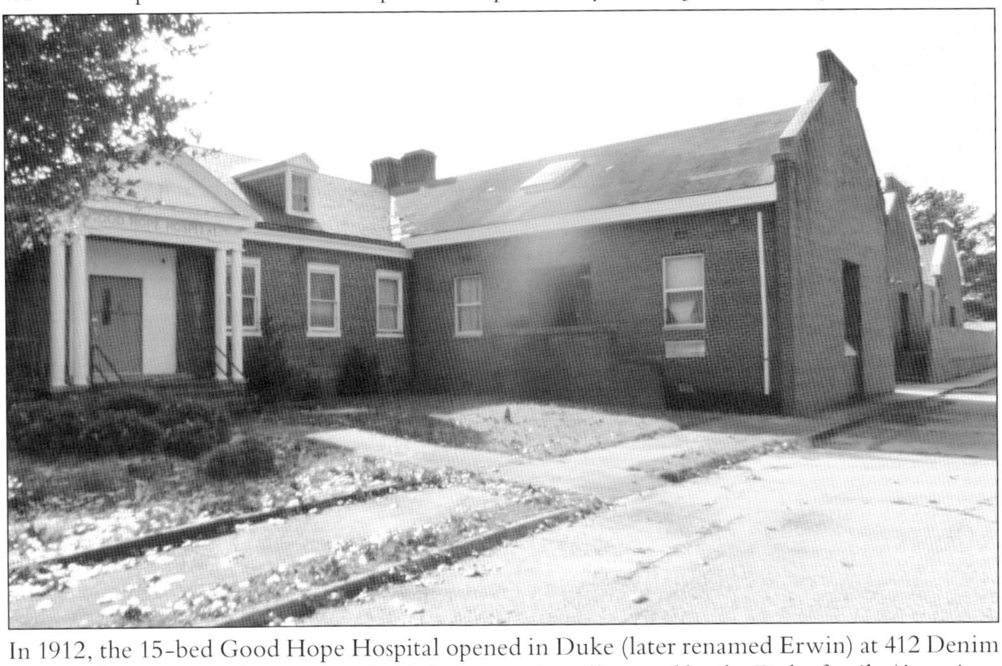

In 1912, the 15-bed Good Hope Hospital opened in Duke (later renamed Erwin) at 412 Denim Drive. The town was the outgrowth of a large textile mill owned by the Duke family (American Tobacco Company). Erwin is just north of the lost town of Averasborough. Good Hope closed in 2006 after a competing CON was approved and another hospital was built (instead of the replacement for Good Hope) in nearby Lillington.

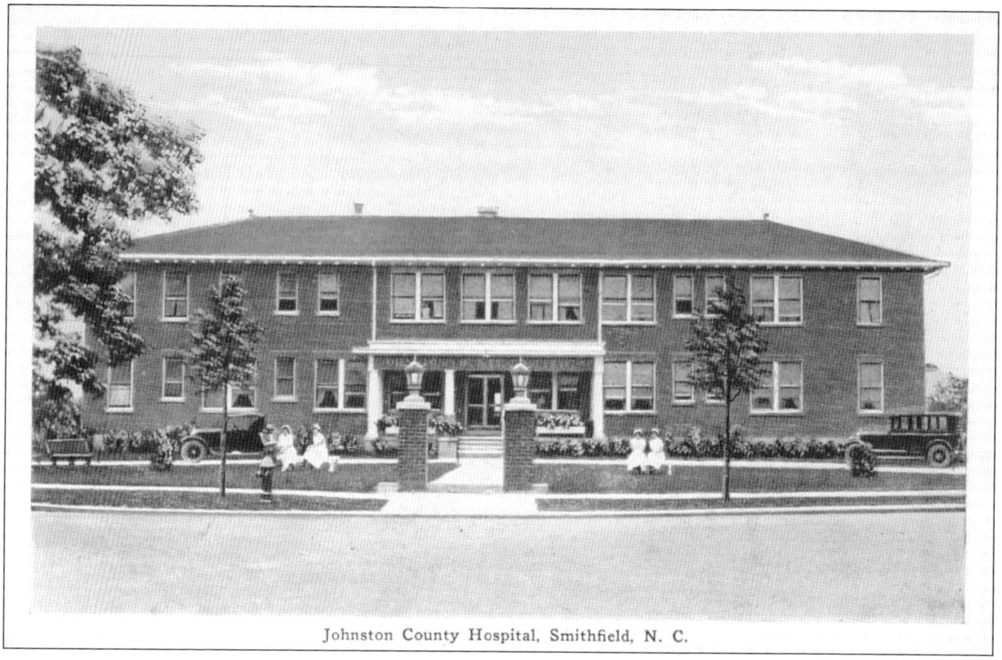

In 1920, the 15-bed Smithfield Memorial Hospital, also known as the Johnston County Hospital, opened with doctors Carl V. Tyner, Thel Hooks, and L.D. Wharton as the physicians.

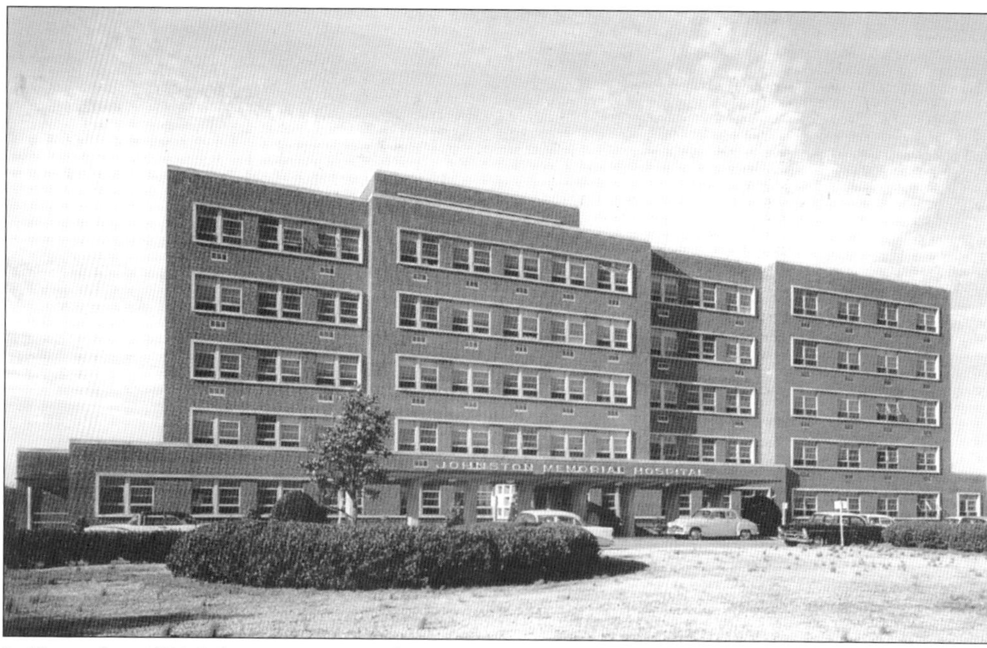

In December 1951, Johnston Memorial Hospital opened. The county voters approved borrowing $275,000 with Hill-Burton funding, and state funds made up the balance of the $1.25 million cost for the 100-bed hospital. Later rebranded Johnston Health, the organization in 2008 added a freestanding emergency department to the outpatient surgery center in Clayton. In 2013, the hospital joined UNC Health Care, and the facility at Clayton was expanded into a full-service 50-bed hospital.

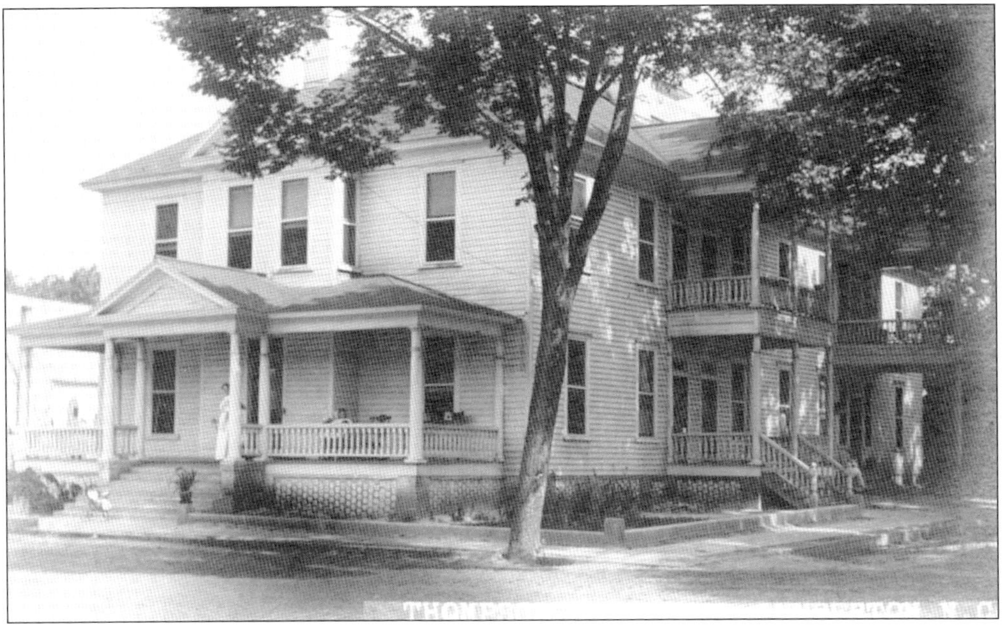

The Thompson Memorial Hospital, Robeson County's first, was established in 1906 by Dr. Neill Archie Thompson. In 1923, the hospital reported 25 beds. This building was destroyed by fire in 1924. A replacement opened in 1925. (Durwood Barbour Collection, Wilson Library, UNC-Chapel Hill.)

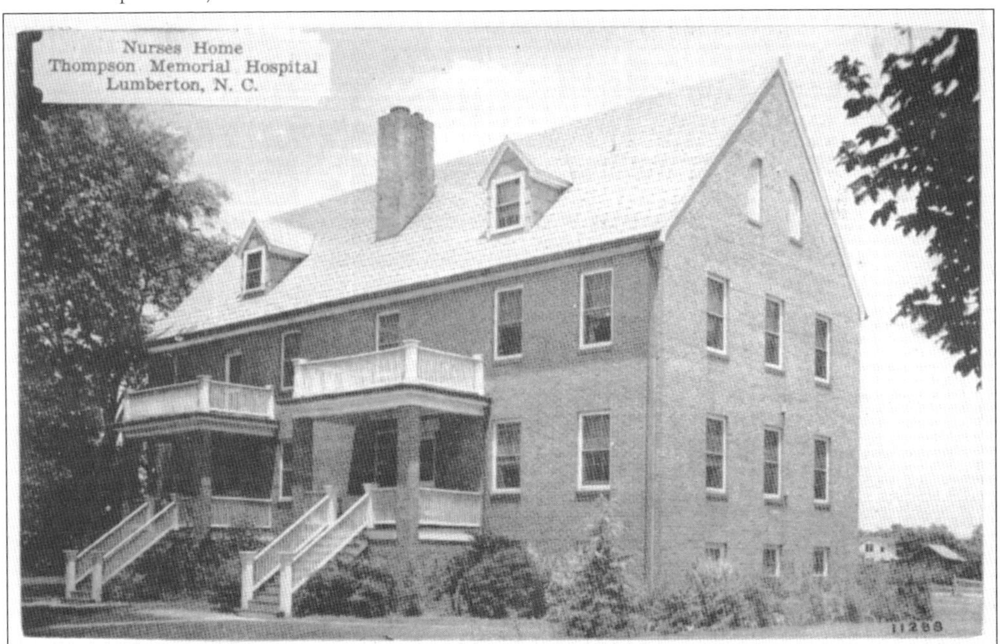

Most nursing education programs of the time included a nurses' residence at or near the sponsor hospital. In the early 20th century, nursing education programs were part classroom lectures and part apprenticeship. The nursing education program closed and transitioned to the local community college in 1966. The Thompson Memorial Hospital Nurses Home in Lumberton was adjacent to the hospital.

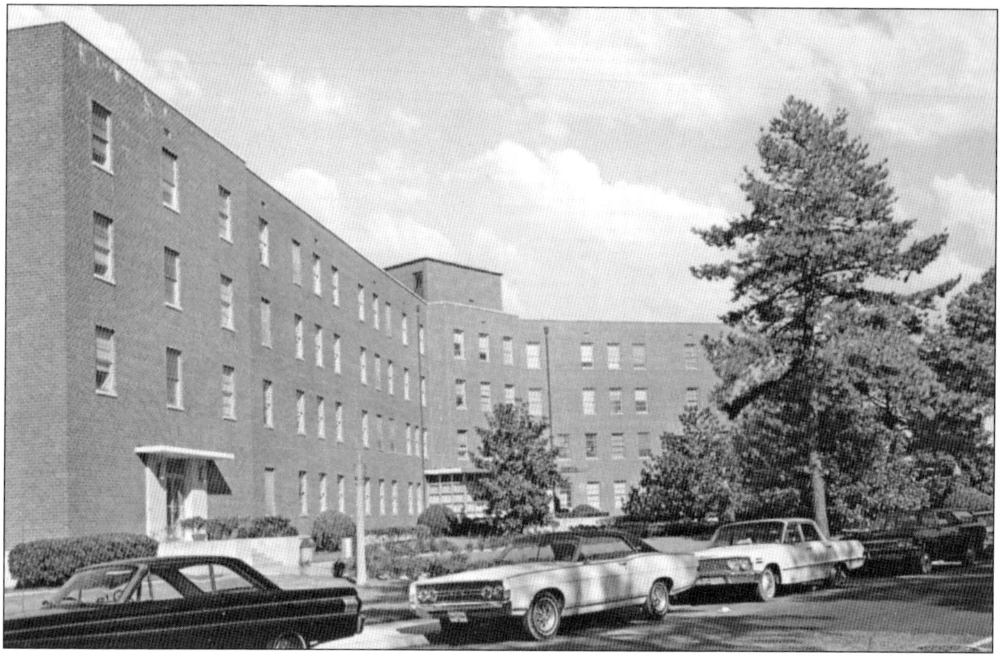

Robeson County Memorial Hospital opened as a 140-bed hospital in Lumberton in August 1953. By 1960, the name was changed to reflect the region served—Southeastern General Hospital. Today, known as Southeastern Regional Medical Center, this 452-bed hospital serves Robeson County and the surrounding region.

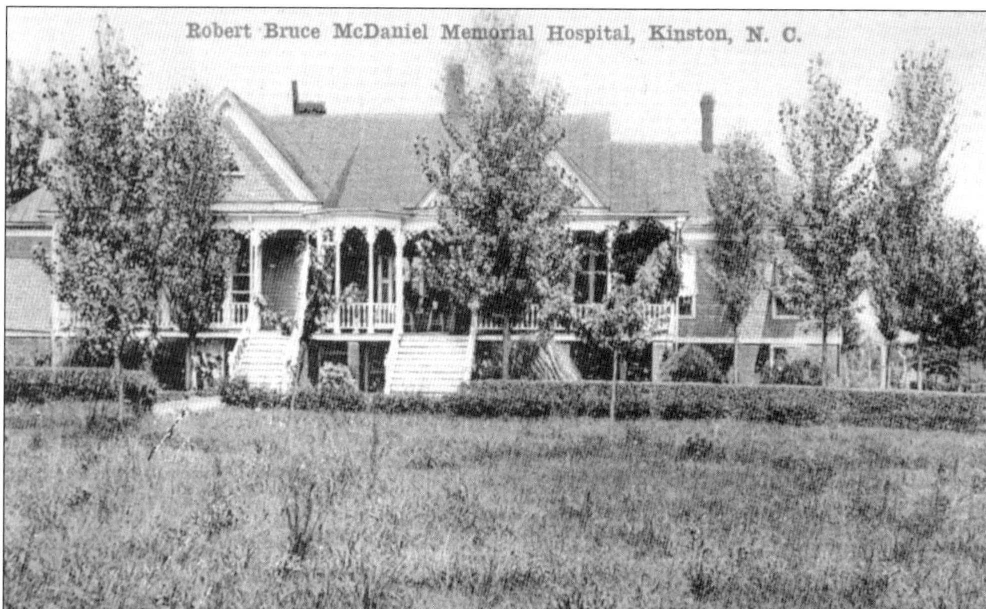

One of the state's first hospitals, Robert Bruce McDaniel Memorial Hospital, opened in 1905 on East Gordon Street. The J.A. McDaniel family donated the hospital property in memory of their son, Robert Bruce, who succumbed to an illness. The two principal physicians were Dr. J.M. Parrott and Dr. W.T. Parrott. In 1914, the brothers acquired the hospital outright and renamed it for their mother as Elisabeth Waters Parrott Memorial Hospital.

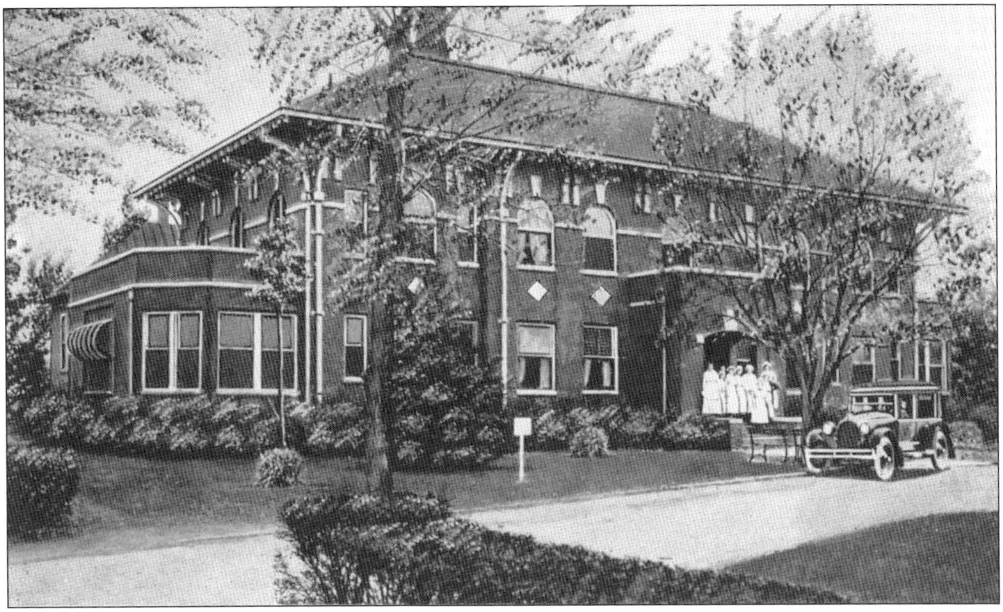

Dr. W.T. Parrott traveled to Germany to study with Dr. W.K. Roentgen, inventor of the X-ray. Dr. Parrott built the first X-ray machine in North Carolina but lost his left hand from radiation overexposure. Parrott Memorial Hospital was sold to Lenoir County in 1966. Along with Memorial General, both hospitals operated under one administration until they closed in 1973, with all patients moving to a newly built Lenoir Memorial Hospital.

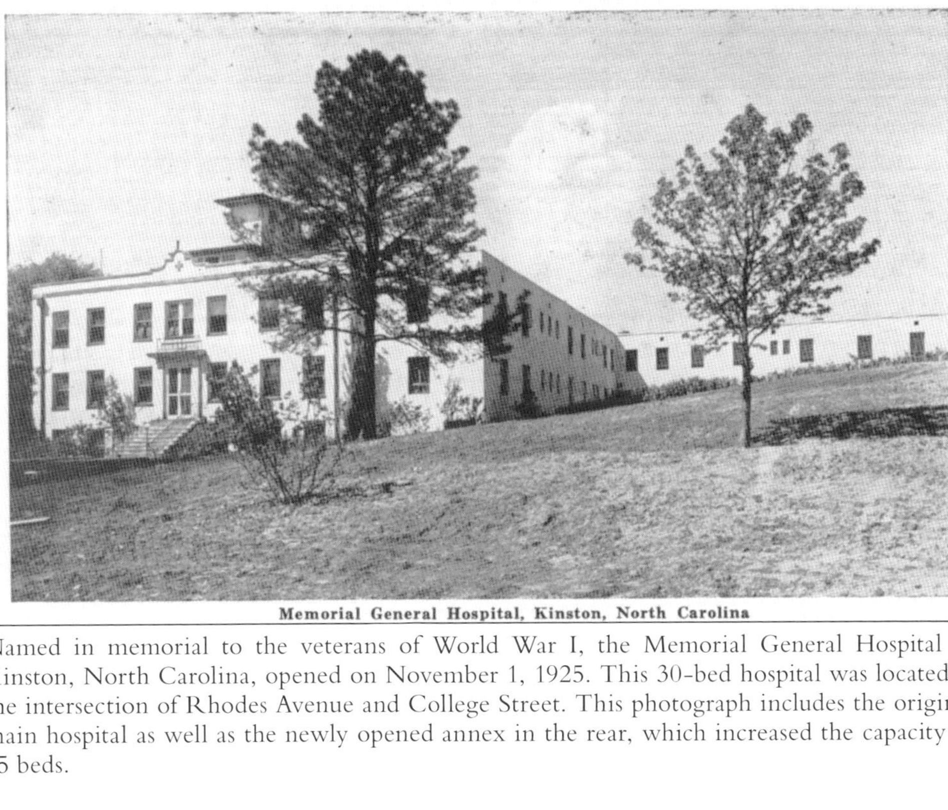

Memorial General Hospital, Kinston, North Carolina

Named in memorial to the veterans of World War I, the Memorial General Hospital in Kinston, North Carolina, opened on November 1, 1925. This 30-bed hospital was located at the intersection of Rhodes Avenue and College Street. This photograph includes the original main hospital as well as the newly opened annex in the rear, which increased the capacity to 75 beds.

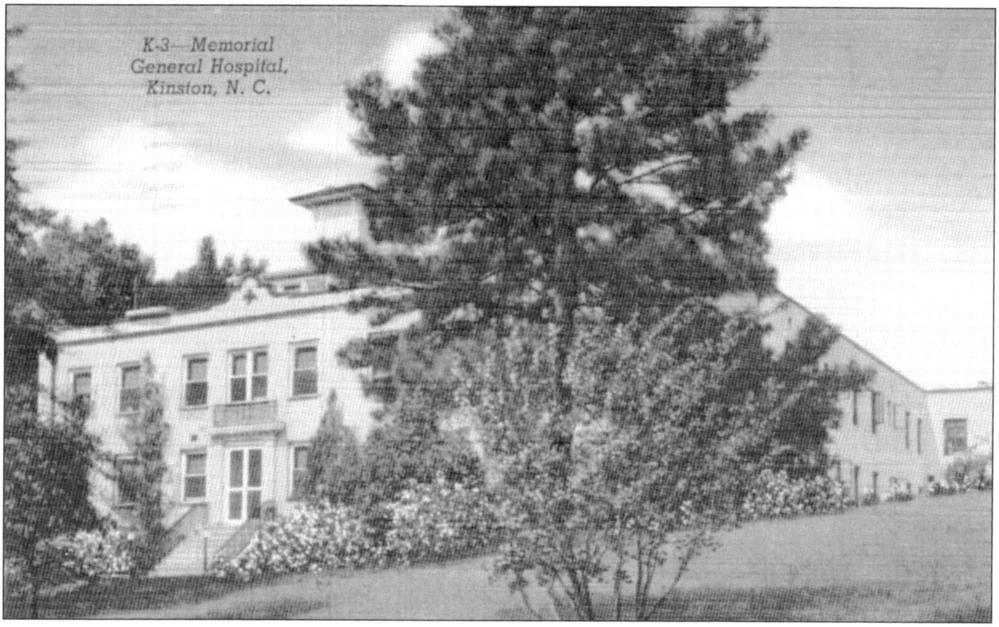

By the mid-1930s, both Memorial General Hospital as well as the crosstown Parrott Memorial Hospital struggled as an economic depression gripped the United States. Both nursing programs closed in 1932, although the nursing program at Memorial General reopened in 1937. It operated along with the Parrott Memorial Hospital, serving the citizens of the Kinston area.

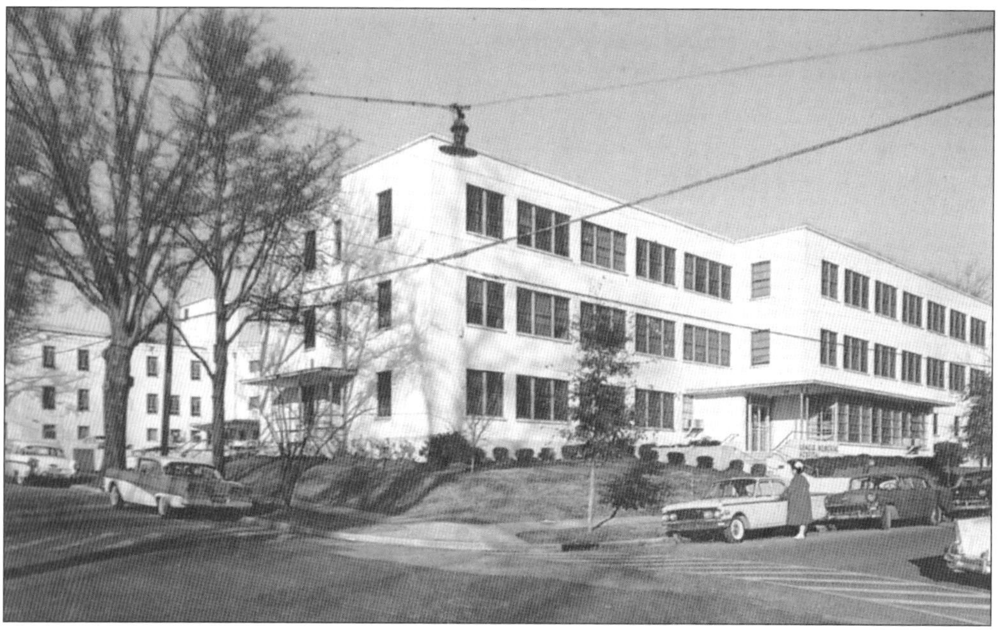

The owners donated the 125-bed Memorial General Hospital to Lenoir County in 1953 so that a bond issue could provide for extensive renovation and increased bed capacity. The hospital name was changed to Lenoir Memorial Hospital. Along with Parrott Memorial Hospital, the two hospitals served the community until a replacement consolidated health care facility, Lenoir Memorial Hospital, opened in the area on July 7, 1973. Today, the hospital is known as UNC Lenoir Health Care.

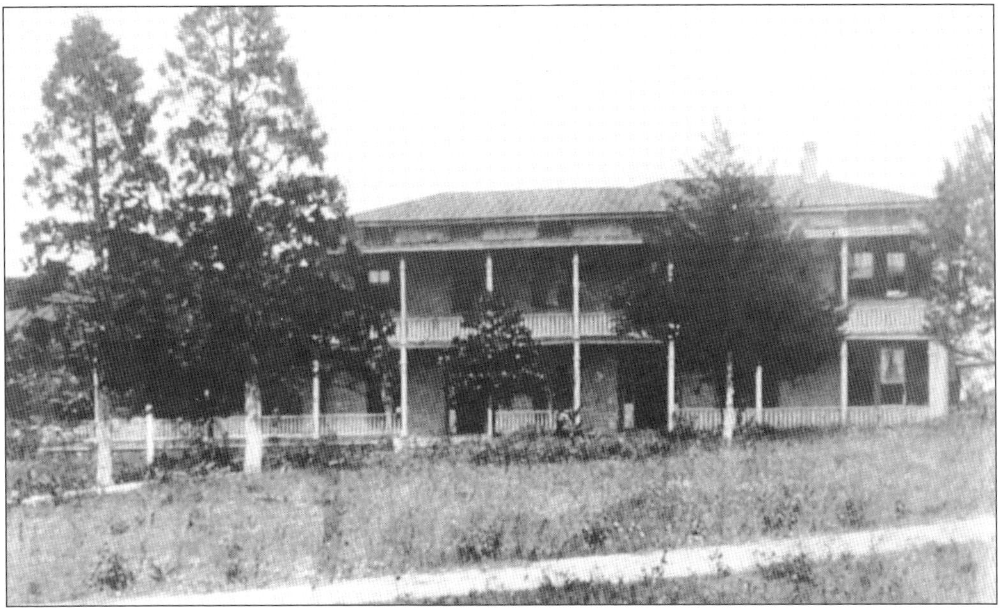

Authorized by the North Carolina General Assembly, the City-County Hospital opened in 1881 in Wilmington. Accessible by horse or a plank sidewalk for those on foot, it was intended to serve the citizens for the foreseeable future. However, it was beset by multiple problems ranging from inadequate funding to poor construction. The facility was replaced by the James Walker Memorial Hospital some 20 years later.

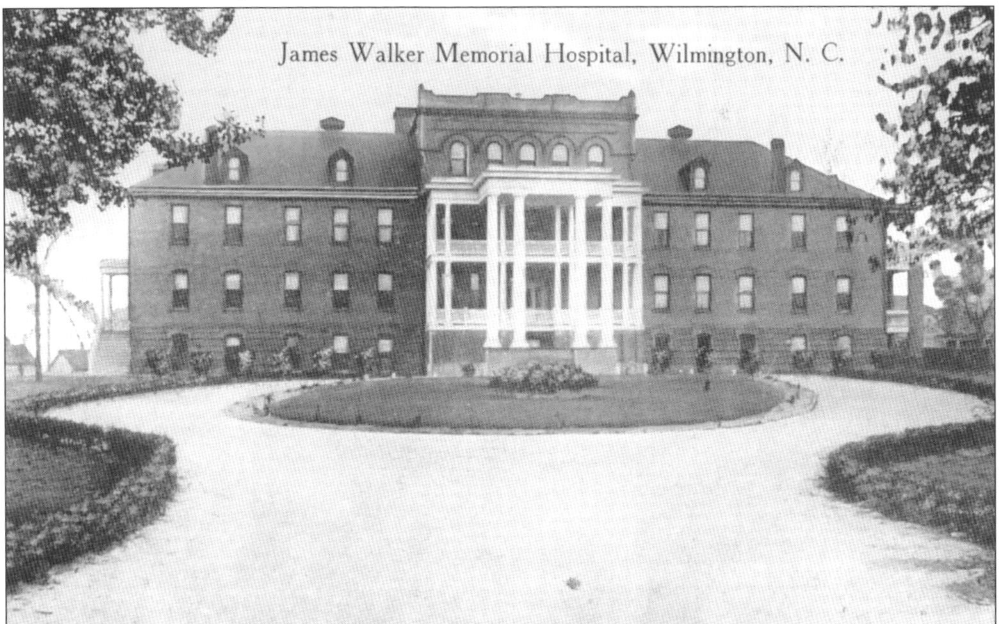

James Walker was a stonemason, contractor, and builder. He came to Wilmington after being awarded the contract in 1856 to build the US Marine Hospital there. One of his later projects included the Western North Carolina Sanatorium. His final project, the James Walker Memorial Hospital, opened in 1901, less than three months after his death. This hospital replaced the City-County Hospital.

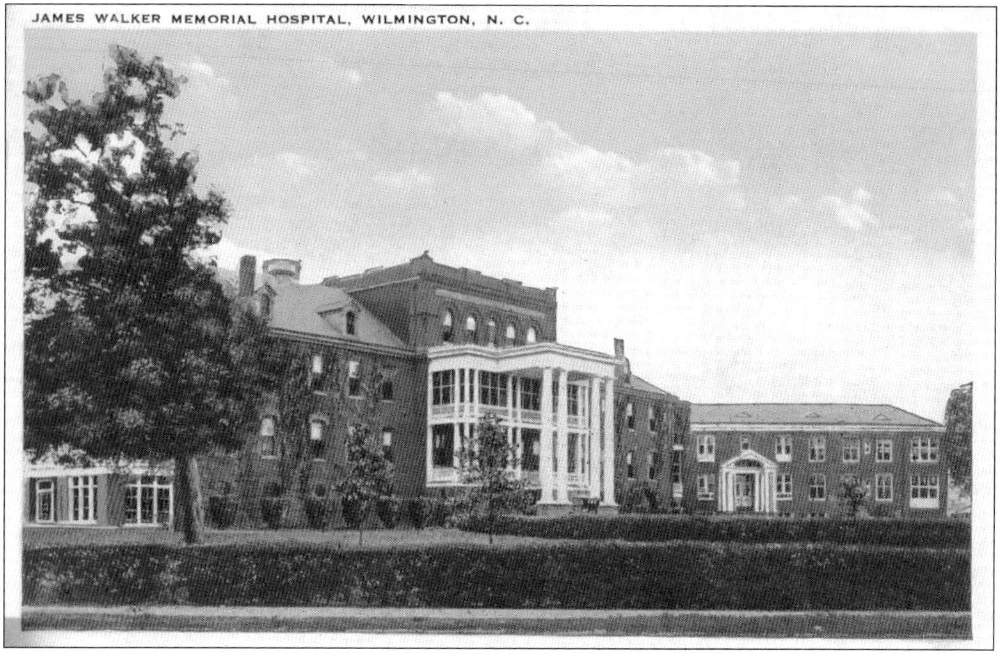

Pictured is a view of the James Walker Memorial Hospital with the south wing addition. By 1923, the 150-bed hospital identified Dr. Bahnson Weathers as the resident physician. The last addition to the James Walker Memorial Hospital took it to 300 beds. This included "wards for blacks," a dispensary, nurses' quarters, a contagious ward, and a maternity and children's ward.

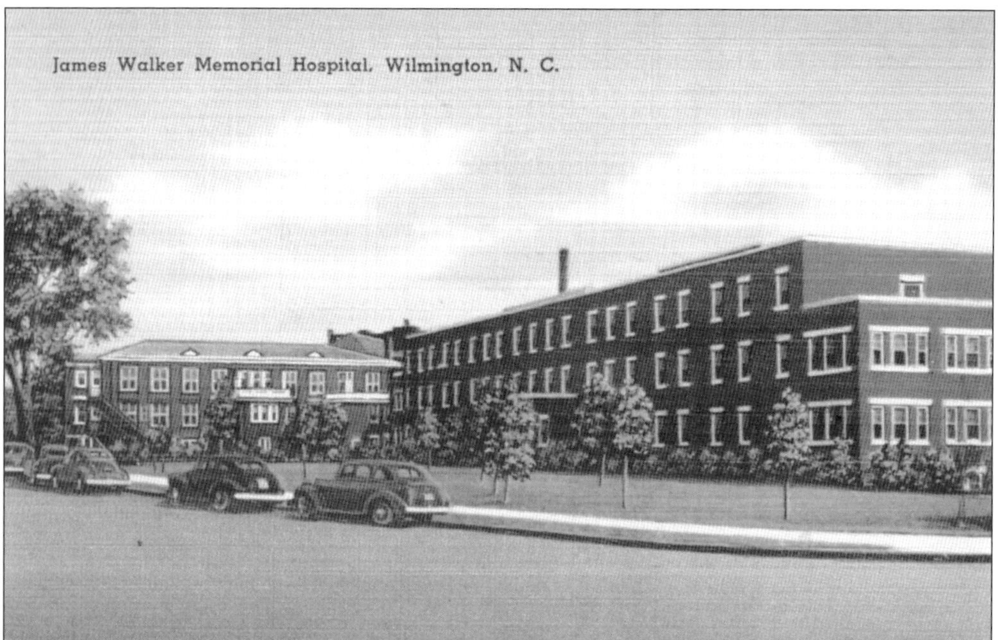

By 1947, the hospital building had a series of additions but those were outdated. Requests for public financial support was repeatedly denied. In 1957, four physicians built Cape Fear Memorial Hospital at the site of the old sanatorium.

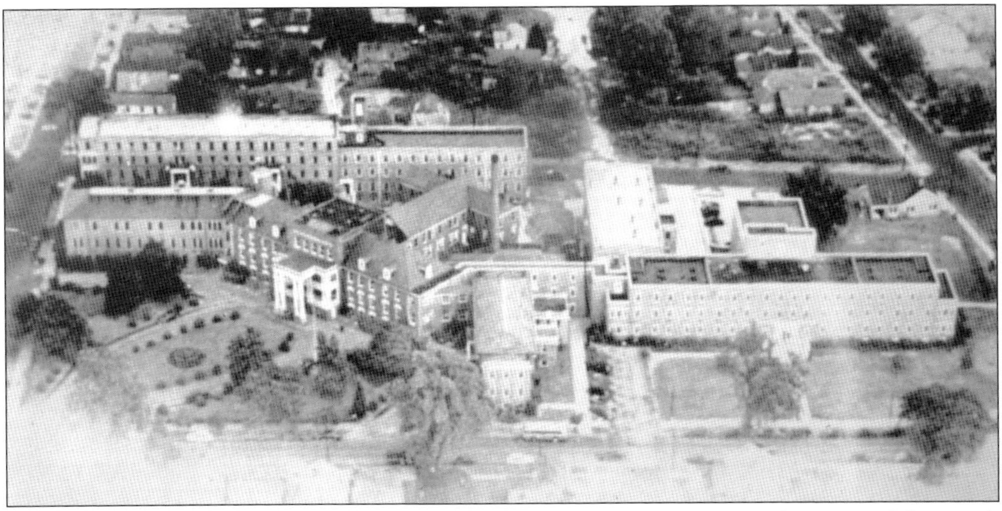

By the late 1950s, James Walker Memorial Hospital was a massive complex (one of the state's largest) but was plagued by antiquated plumbing and electrical issues. A second referendum passed in 1961 to build a new consolidated hospital. In 1966, New Hanover Memorial Hospital opened, and the patients at Community and James Walker Memorial Hospitals were transferred to the new hospital, with James Walker Memorial and Community closing. (New Hanover County Public Library.)

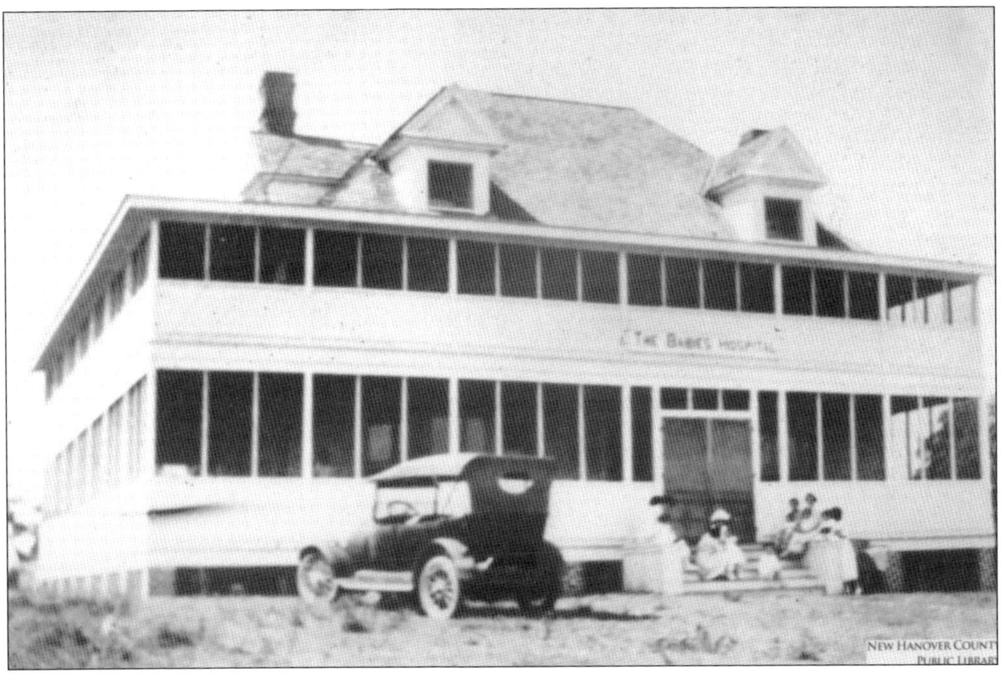

Babies Hospital, near Wrightsville Sound, was opened in 1920 to take advantage of the "air's curative powers" by Dr. J. Buren Sidbury, who was the second pediatrician in North Carolina. Dr. Sidbury's hospital was the only North Carolina pediatric hospital until Duke Hospital opened in 1930. The original wooden structure (pictured here) burned in 1927. Luckily, there were no injuries. In 1928, a replacement hospital opened across the street. (New Hanover County Public Library.)

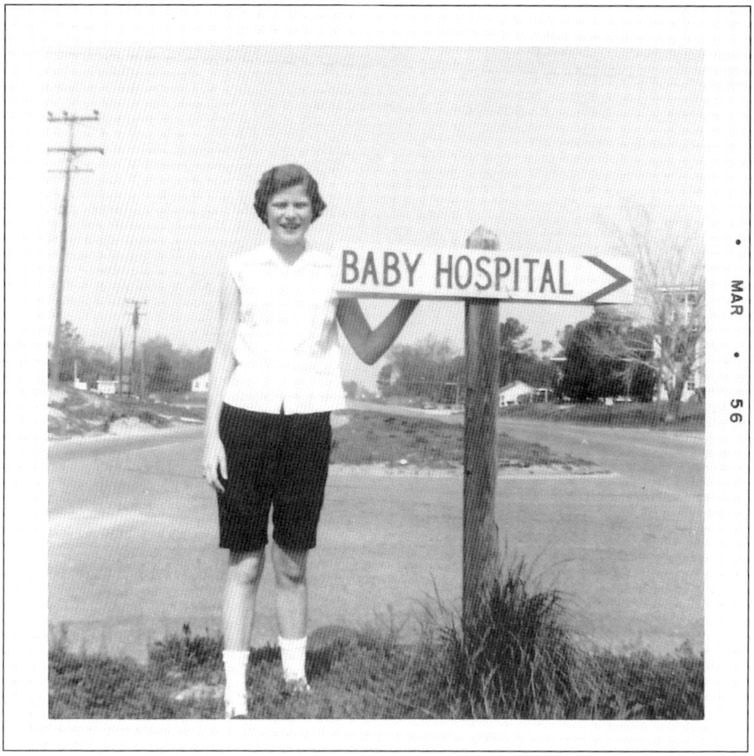
BABY HOSPITAL
MAR • 56

A nurse who worked at the Babies Hospital is shown here as she prepares for her seasonal duties at the hospital. This photograph is dated March 1956. While the hospital began to operate year-round in 1939, the seasonal nature drew far more patients in the summer than at any other point, requiring seasonal staff to augment the permanent staff. (Photograph provided by Sonia O'Brien.)

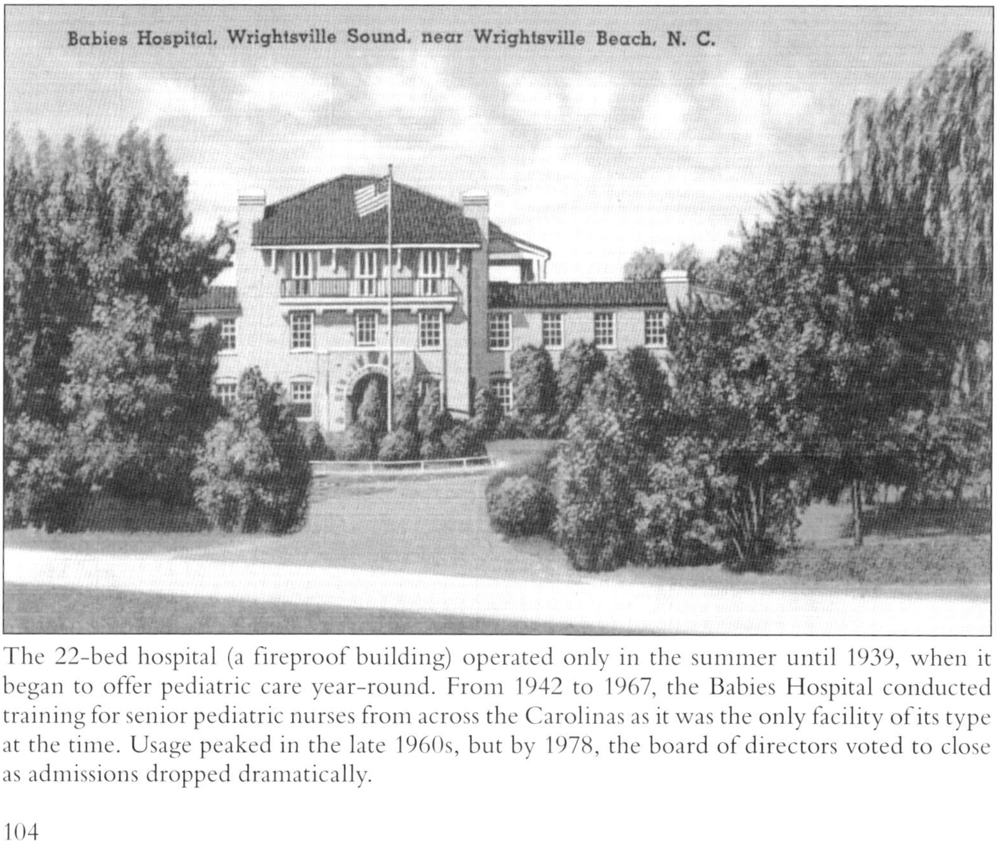
Babies Hospital, Wrightsville Sound, near Wrightsville Beach, N. C.

The 22-bed hospital (a fireproof building) operated only in the summer until 1939, when it began to offer pediatric care year-round. From 1942 to 1967, the Babies Hospital conducted training for senior pediatric nurses from across the Carolinas as it was the only facility of its type at the time. Usage peaked in the late 1960s, but by 1978, the board of directors voted to close as admissions dropped dramatically.

Located at 221 North Front Street, the 50-bed Bulluck Hospital was the first North Carolina hospital to hire a female physician—Dr. Annie T. Smith. The hospital opened in downtown on September 1, 1922, and reported Dr. R.H. Davis as the PIC in 1923. It closed in 1944. Today, the building is used by Wilmington Downtown, Inc. (New Hanover County Library.)

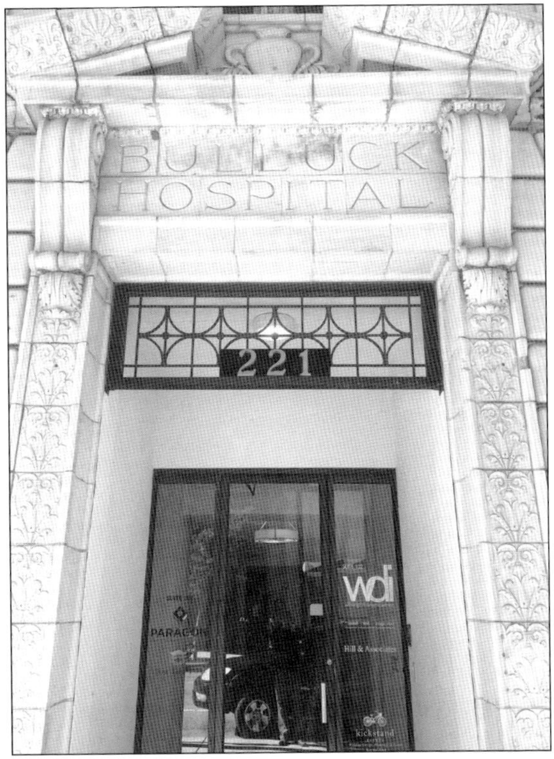

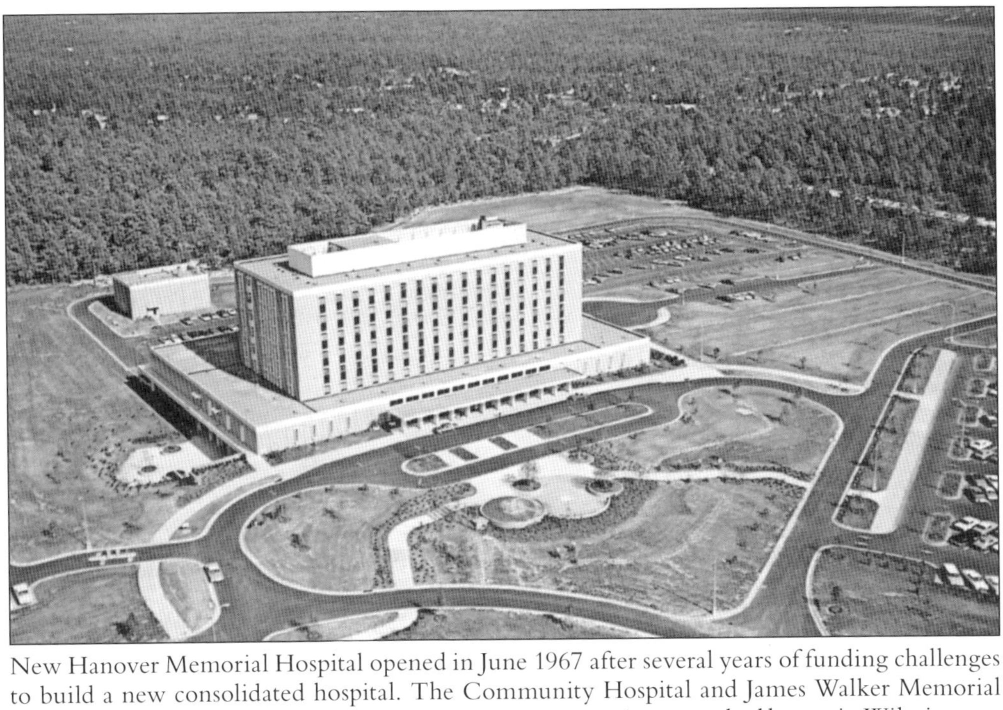

New Hanover Memorial Hospital opened in June 1967 after several years of funding challenges to build a new consolidated hospital. The Community Hospital and James Walker Memorial Hospital closed, and patients were moved to New Hanover. A new era had begun in Wilmington. In 1998, Cape Fear Memorial was merged into the system. Today, the New Hanover Memorial Hospital anchors the 855-bed New Hanover Regional Health Care System.

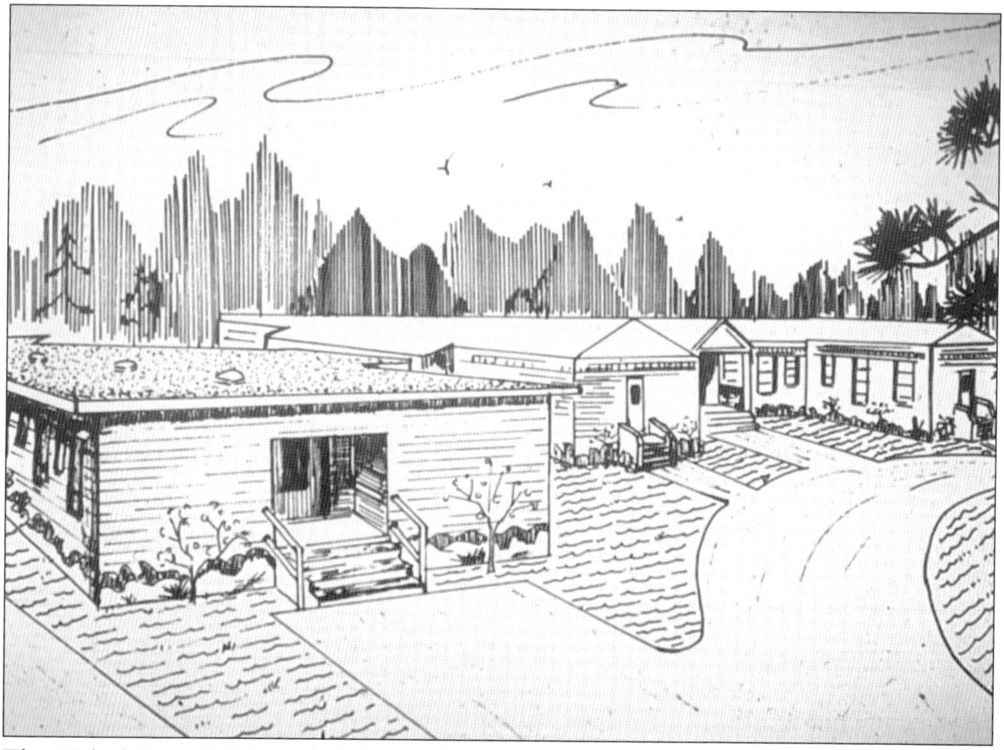

The 32-bed Wessell Tuberculosis Sanatorium was established in 1951 with Dr. Robert Boyd Rodman as the physician in charge. Located at 5301 Wrightsville Avenue, it later closed but was reopened as the 40-bed Cape Fear Memorial Hospital on August 6, 1957. The hospital was sold to Hospital Corporation of America before being acquired in 1998 by New Hanover Regional Medical Center. Today, the building serves as a satellite facility for the main campus, providing dedicated inpatient and outpatient orthopedic care.

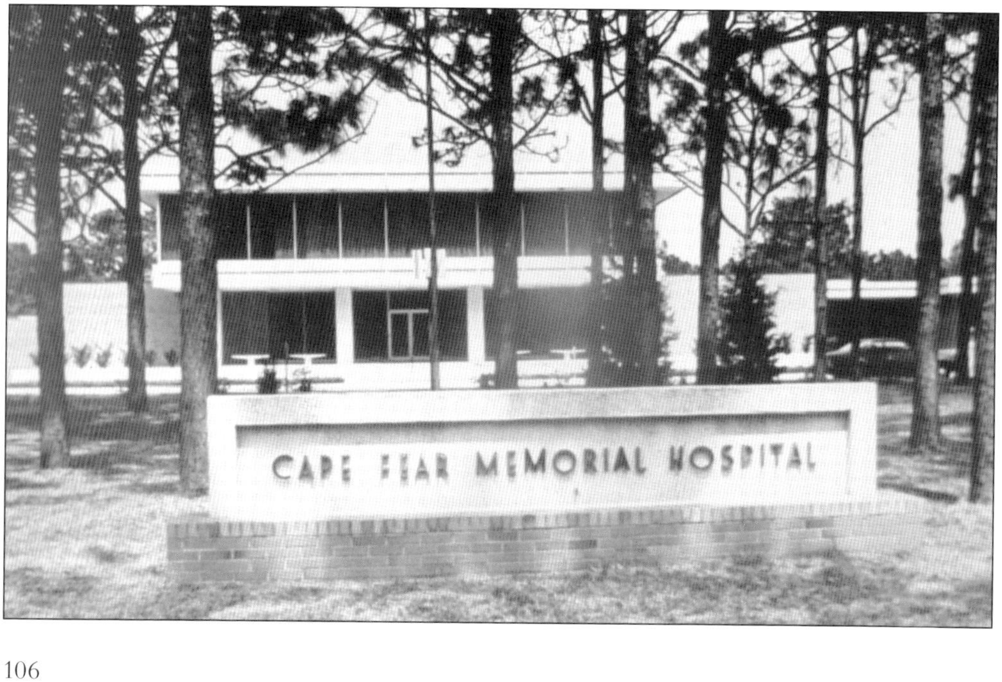

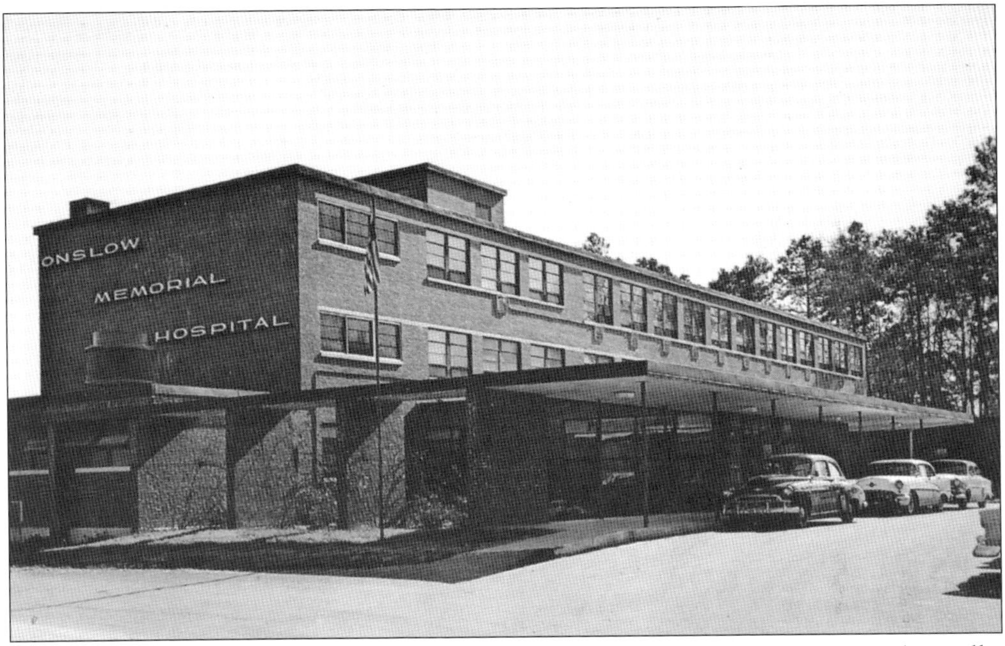

In 1944, the 60-bed Onslow County Hospital opened at 317 Western Boulevard in Jacksonville. Today, Onslow Memorial is a 162-bed hospital.

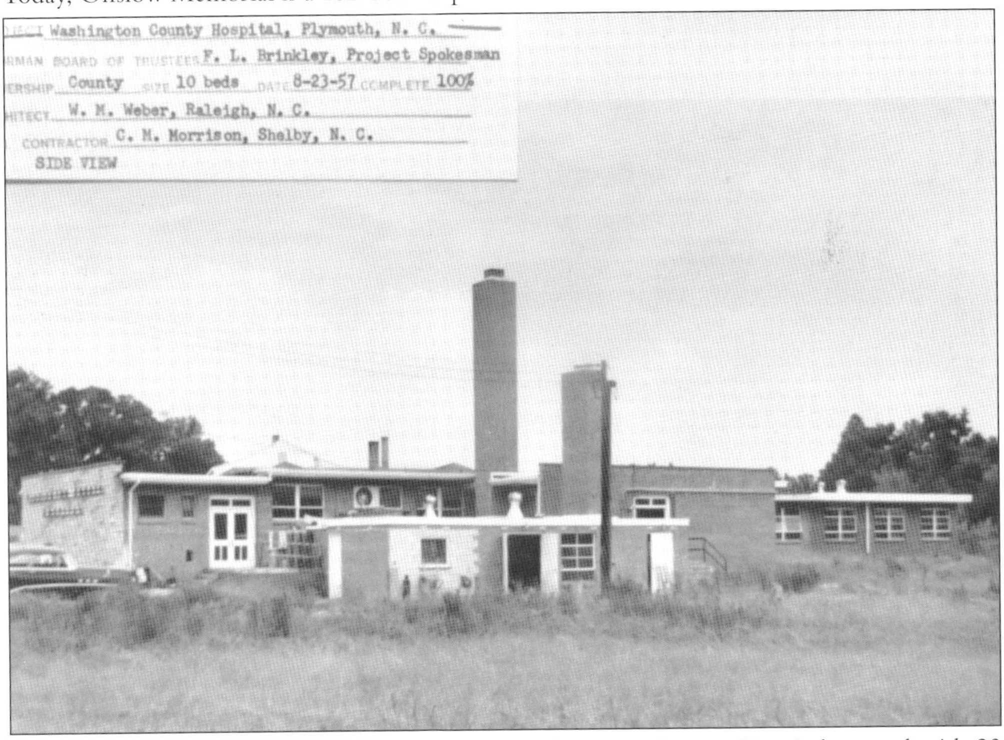

In 1950, with the aid of Hill-Burton funding, Washington County Hospital opened with 23 beds. Today, licensed as a 49-bed hospital, Washington County Hospital is operated as a 25-bed CAH located on US Highway 64 in Plymouth. The hospital is owned and operated by Rural Community Hospitals of America. (North Carolina State Archives.)

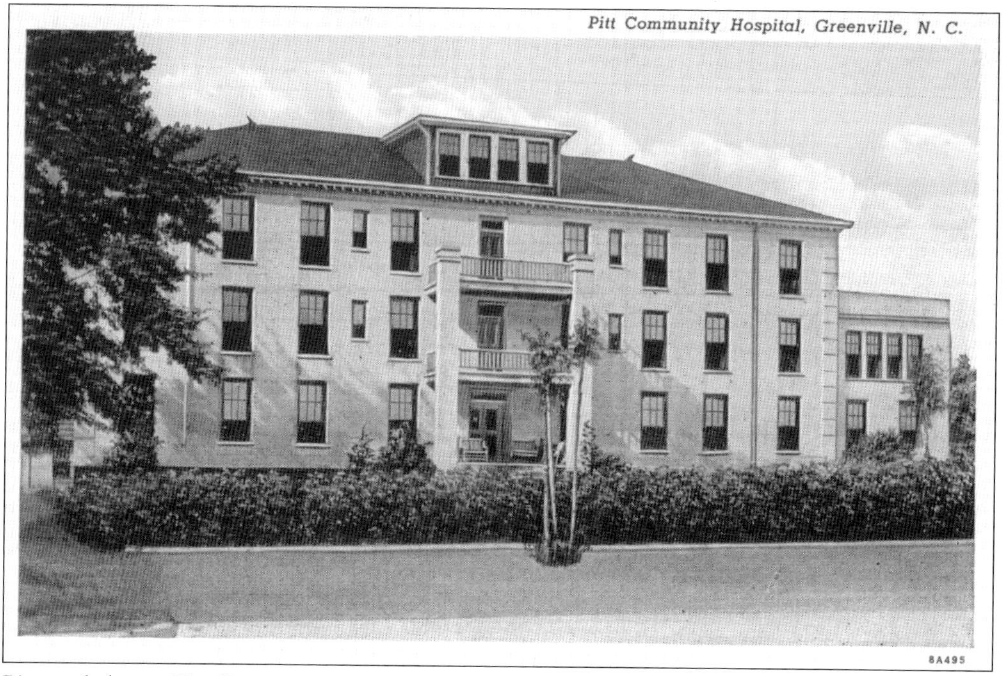

Pictured above, Pitt Community Hospital (also called Greenville Community) opened in 1924 at the corner of Johnston and Woodlawn Streets with 42 beds (41 for whites, one for blacks). In September 1923, during construction, a temporary hospital opened at 210 East Fifth Street, above a hardware store. In 1935, the hospital split into two divisions with Pitt Community operating a clinic and taking the surgical patients and Pitt General Hospital serving the charity care patients (in the same building). Creation of the two divisions was done to take advantage of Duke Endowment funds. Pitt General absorbed the Pitt Community assets in 1940. Pitt General closed when Pitt Memorial opened in 1951 with the county purchasing the assets. Pictured below, Pitt County Memorial Hospital opened in January 1951. The 120-bed hospital included a 30-bed "colored ward."

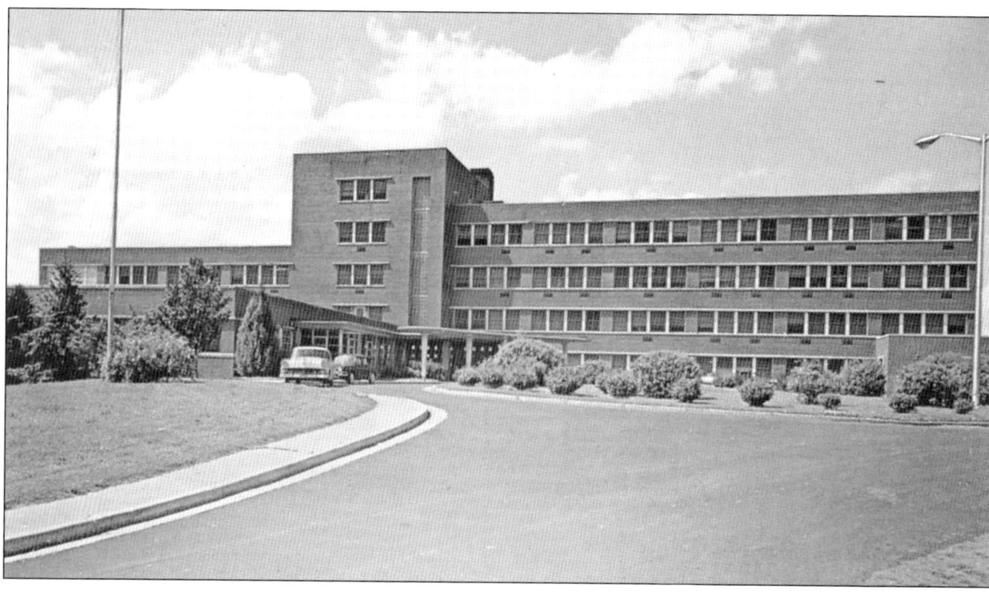

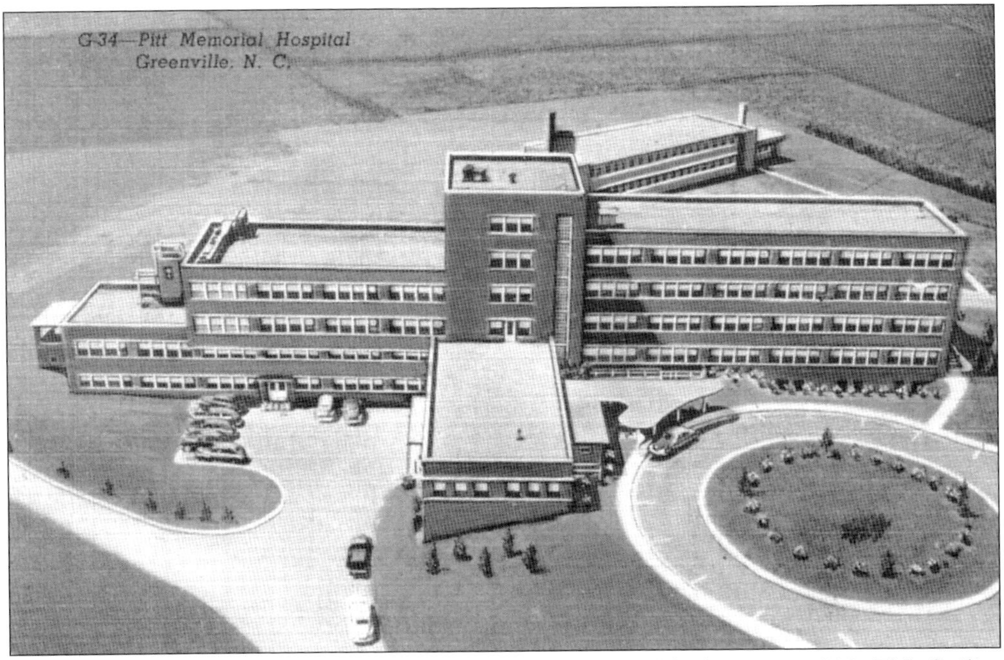

The rear patient wing was added in 1958, bringing the total bed count to 205. This facility would be replaced in 1977 by the hospital at its current location in west Greenville, adjacent to the East Carolina University School of Medicine. Today, the hospital has more than 900 beds, and the Vidant Medical Center is the flagship hospital for Vidant Health.

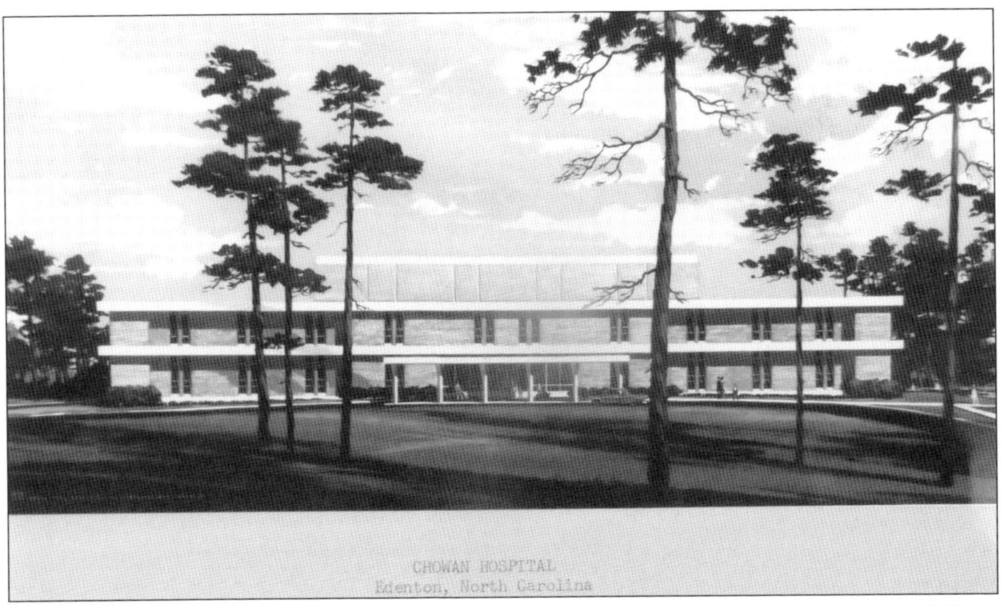

Chowan Hospital opened in 1947. It moved in 1950 and again to its present location in 1970. At one point, the hospital had 49 beds with a 40-bed skilled nursing facility. The hospital joined the University Health System of Eastern Carolina (Vidant Health) in 1998. Today, known as the Vidant Chowan Hospital, the facility is a CAH. (North Carolina State Archives.)

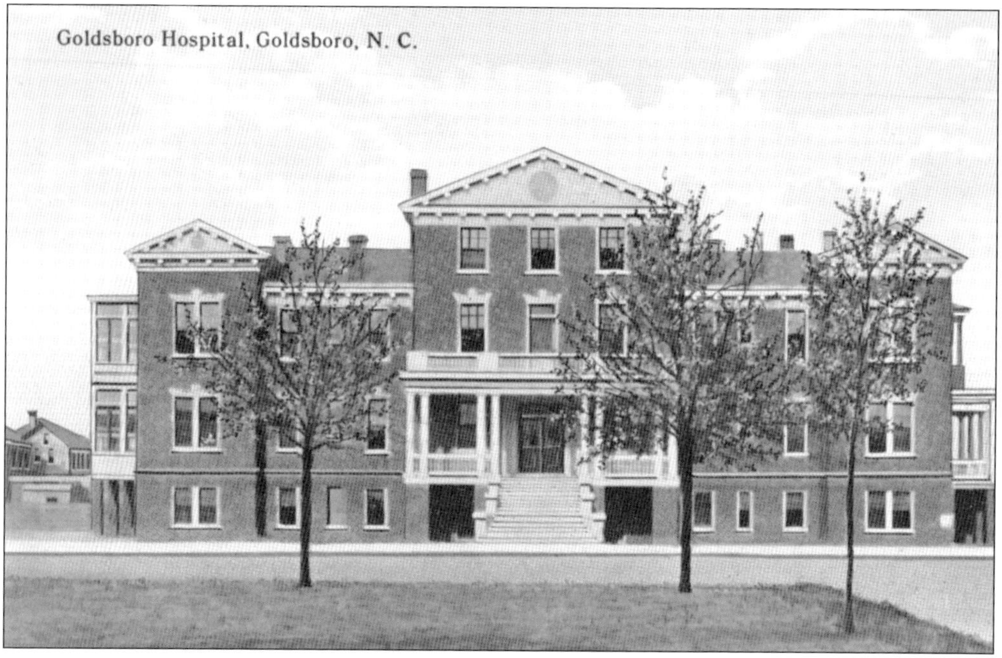

After witnessing the need and lack of help for an injured man in 1894, the pastor for Goldsboro's First Presbyterian Church mobilized his congregation and several prominent citizens to raise money and fund a hospital. Wayne Memorial Hospital opened in 1896. The hospital pictured above was located at the intersection of Ash Street and Herman Street. (Durwood Barbour Collection, Wilson Library, UNC-Chapel Hill.)

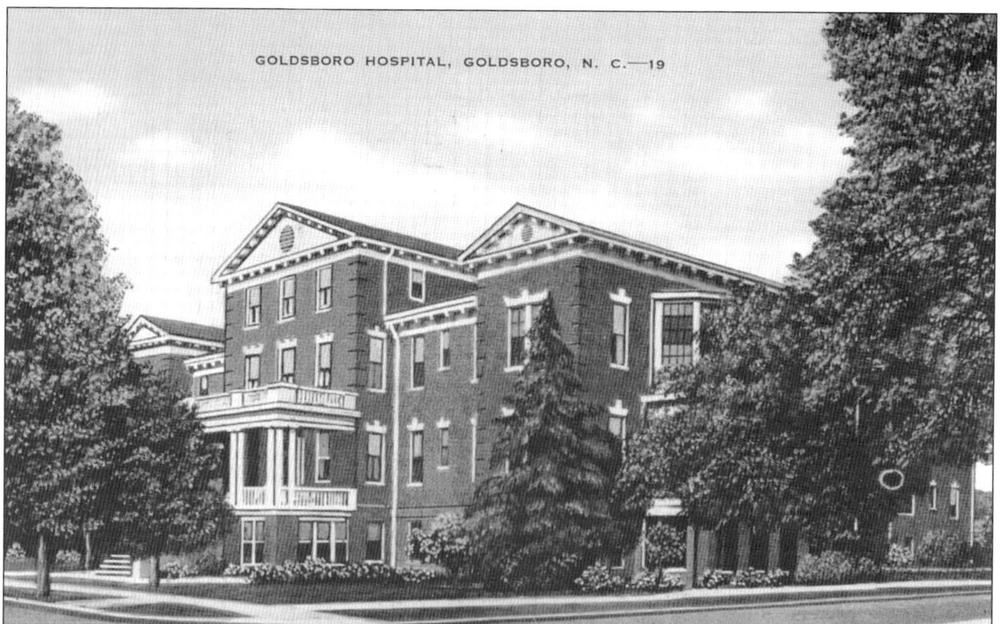

Wayne Memorial Hospital underwent multiple additions before reaching the limits of the available land. The former hospital continues to serve as the Public Health Department.

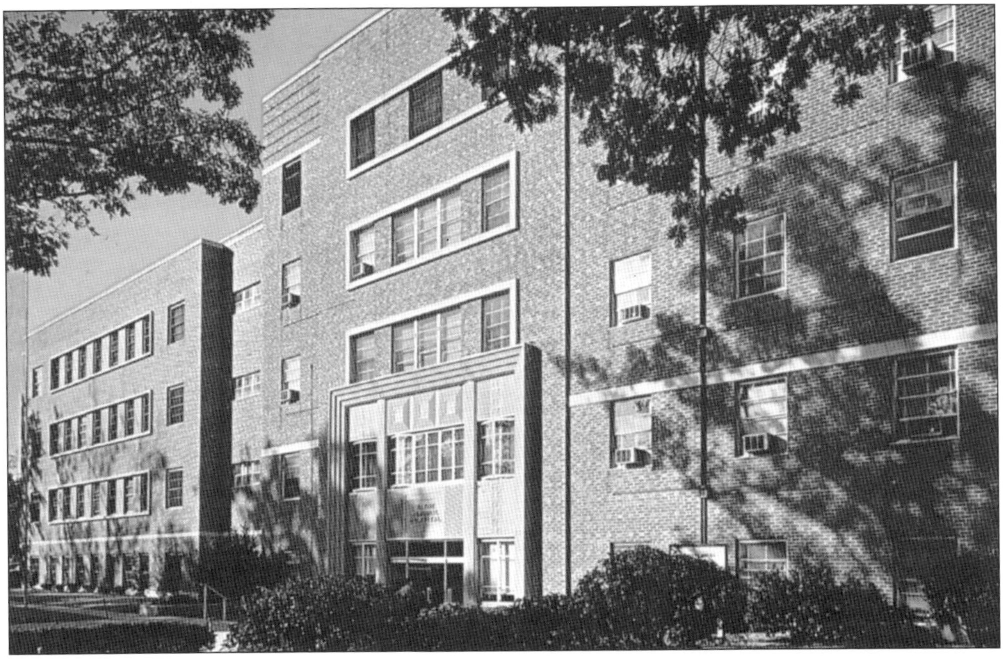

Pictured here, the renovated wing (facing Ash Street) was the last of the Wayne Memorial Hospital additions/renovations in the 1980s. In 1990, a 300-plus-bed replacement hospital was built just north of Highway 70 at 2700 Wayne Memorial Drive. Today, the hospital is part of the UNC Hospitals network and known as UNC Wayne Health Care.

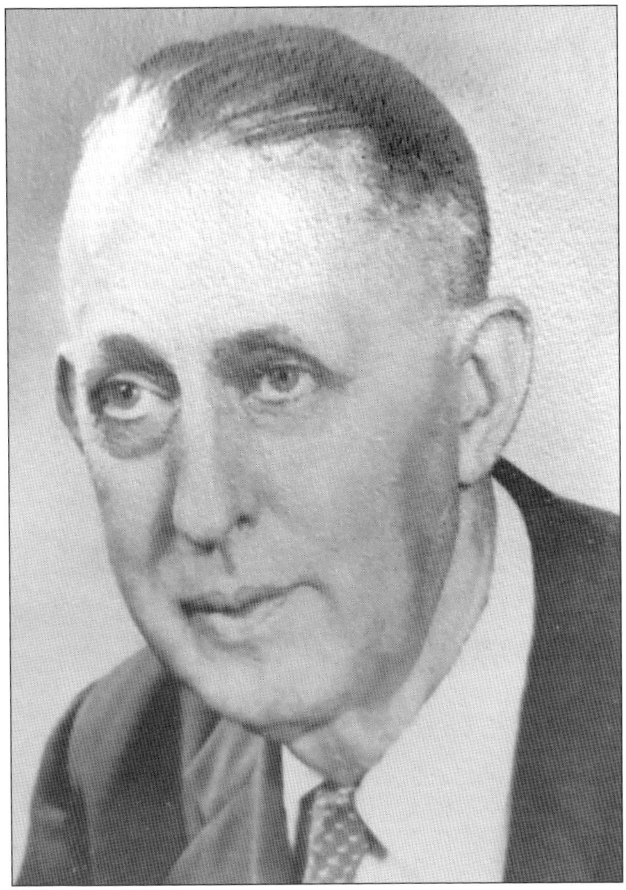

Dr. Claire C. Henderson graduated from the University of North Carolina and arrived in Mt. Olive in 1915, joining Dr. Strosnider as one of the town doctors. In 1949, Dr. Warren H. Crumpler joined Henderson, and they opened the Henderson-Crumpler Clinic (hospital). In 1956, it reported 12 beds and 12 bassinets and operated primarily as a maternity hospital. The hospital function of the clinic ended by the late 1960s.

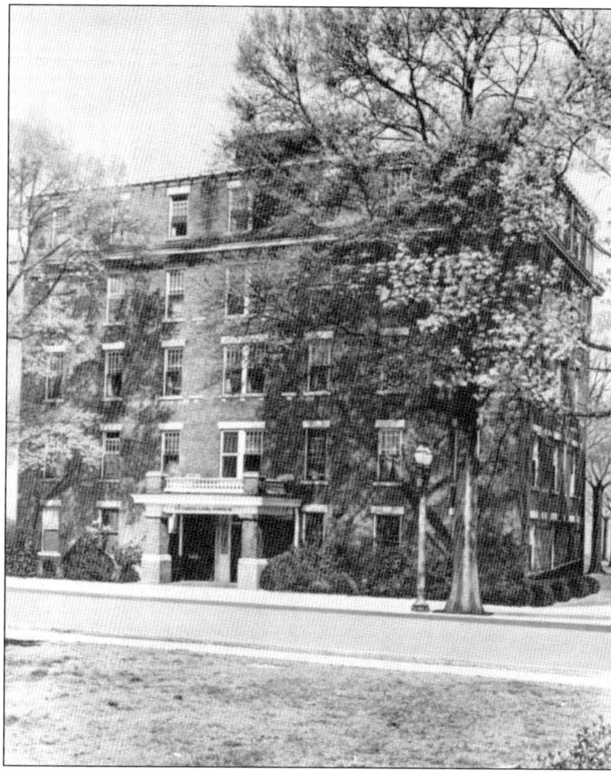

Carolina General Hospital was established in 1919. The 45-bed hospital reported Dr. Paul P. Lane as the physician in charge in 1923. Carolina General briefly merged with Moore-Herring in 1928 but shortly thereafter returned to being operated separately. In 1964, the hospital's assets were purchased, and the facility closed as a part of the transition to the Wilson Memorial Hospital. (Digital NC, Wilson County Public Library.)

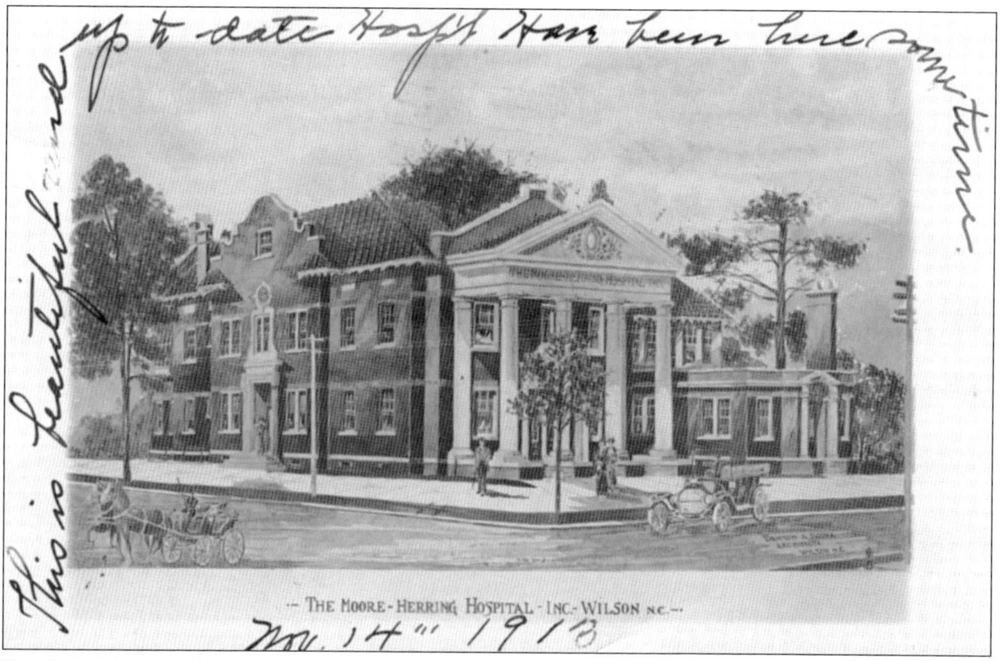
This is beautiful and up to date Hosp't Has been here some time.
— THE MOORE-HERRING HOSPITAL - INC - WILSON NC. —
Nov. 14" 1913

Dr. C.E. Moore left Wilson Sanatorium and, with Dr. Herring, established the Moore-Herring Hospital. The 25-bed hospital was located at the corner of Green and Spring Streets in Wilson in 1913. Dr. B.S. Herring was the physician in charge. (Durwood Barbour Collection, Wilson Library, UNC-Chapel Hill.)

Carolina General Hospital and Moore-Herring Hospital merged in 1928. Less than a year later, the hospitals separated. By 1935, the Moore-Herring Hospital name was changed to Woodard-Herring Hospital (although identified in some materials as Wood-Herring Hospital). (Digital NC, Wilson County Public Library.)

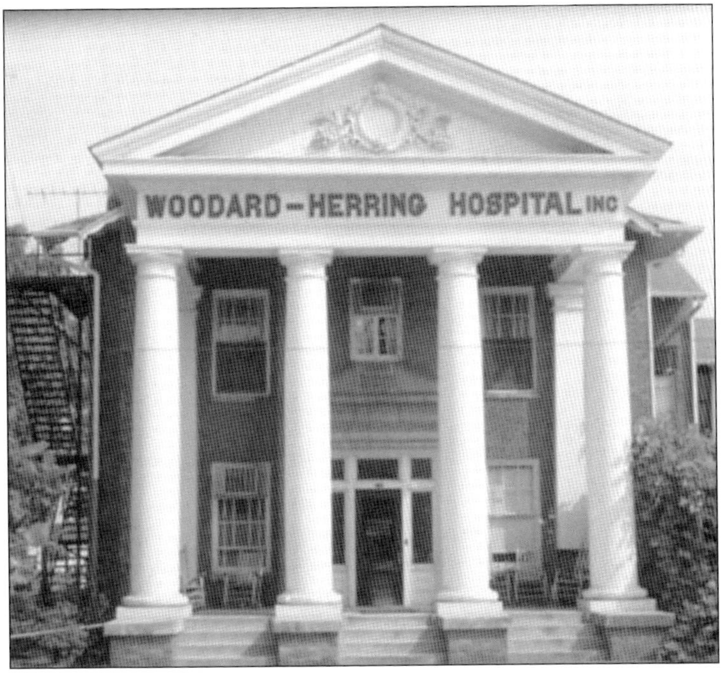

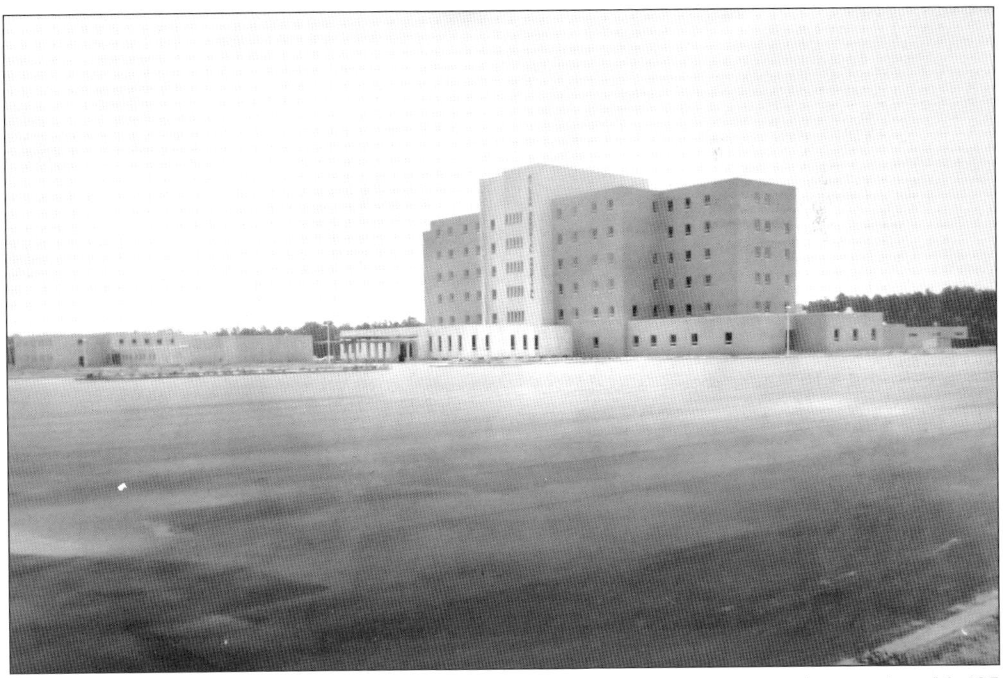

After a failed bond referendum in 1959, a renewed effort in 1960 passed, covering $3.625 million. The local hospitals were purchased as a function of this effort, and the consolidated Wilson Memorial Hospital opened on September 1, 1964, at 1705 Tarboro Street SW, as a 300-bed hospital. It joined the Duke LifePoint Hospital System in 2014. (Digital NC, Wilson County Public Library.)

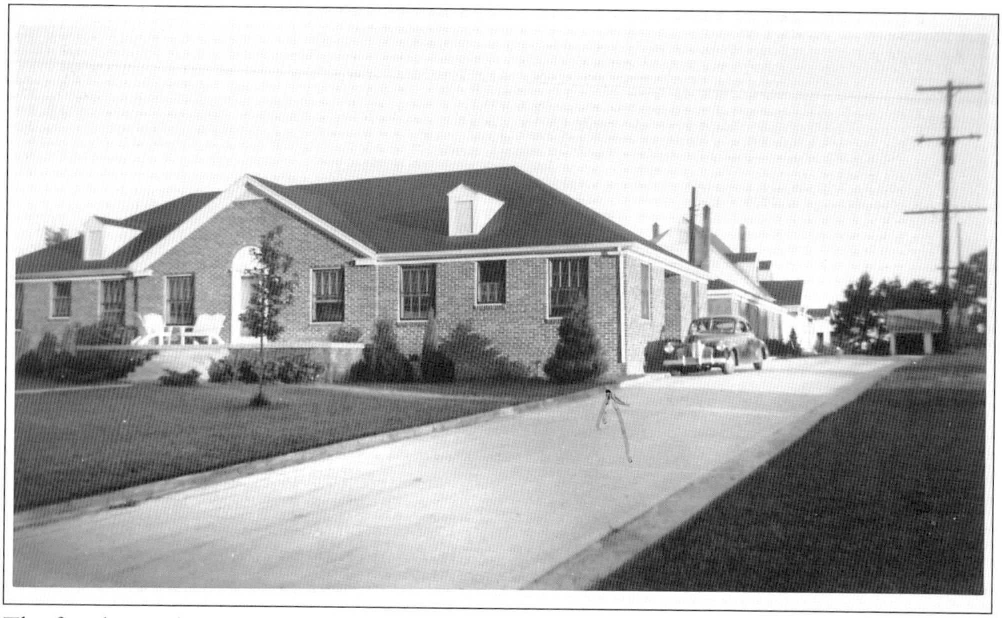

The first hospital in Williamston was the Brown Community Hospital, established in 1939 at 1000 Main Street. Dr. Victor E. Brown owned and managed the private 25-bed hospital. Dr. Brown died January 1960. The facility closed, and the equipment was donated to a hospital in Brazil several years later. Today, the structure is used as an apartment building. (Photograph by Victor Brown Jr.)

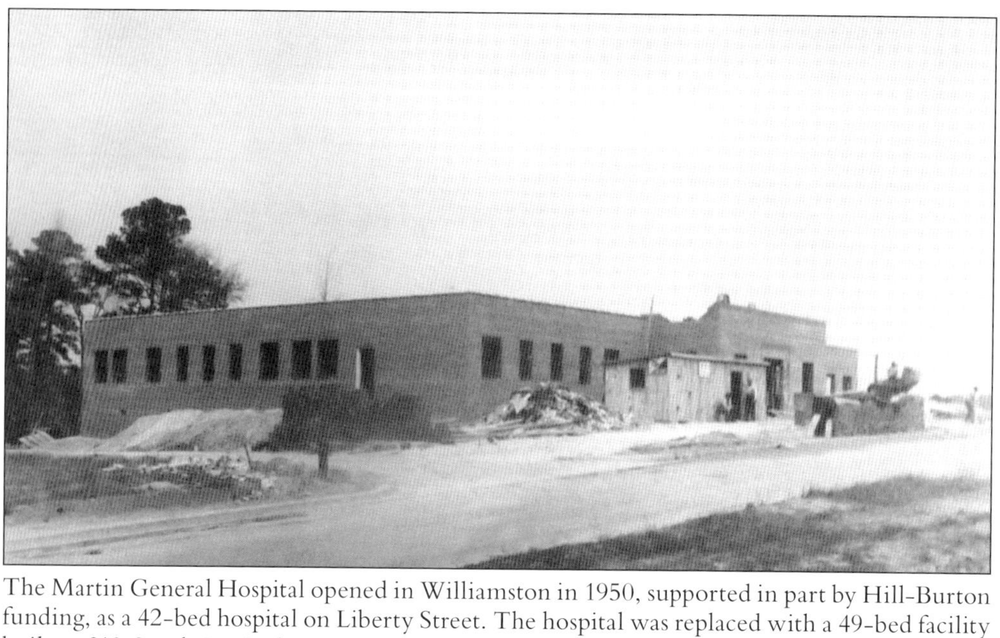

The Martin General Hospital opened in Williamston in 1950, supported in part by Hill-Burton funding, as a 42-bed hospital on Liberty Street. The hospital was replaced with a 49-bed facility built at 310 South McCaskey Road. Today, the hospital is managed by Community Health Care System. (From the Francis Manning Room, Martin Public Library.)

Nine

Medical Schools, Almshouses, Ambulances, and Medical Postcard Artifacts

The sanatoriums, asylums, and hospitals relied on crude and rudimentary tools of medicine at the time. Nevertheless, health care evolved, services and organizations emerged that supported these great institutions, and education became the cornerstone of change for health care. This chapter will explore a sample of these items.

Medical lectures were common at the 300-bed US Marine Hospital at Portsmouth Village before the Civil War. Physicians in training were reviewed at Goldsboro for approval by the Confederate Medical Corps. Between 1865 and 1880, two medical schools opened and closed in Eastern North Carolina. More recently, another opened in Greenville.

The almshouse was a charity-based home, typically for the elderly or orphans. The almshouse was referred to as the "poorhouse" or the "county home" if operated by a local government. The almshouse reflected a need to house a growing number of people who could no earn enough to pay for housing. Larger facilities typically included a physician and an infirmary or hospital.

Ambulances played a significant role in the American Civil War. Following the war, along with the emergence of civilian hospitals and sanatoriums, many included an ambulance service to transport patients to their hospitals. In many cities, surgeons were staffing the ambulance. More recently, the emergency medical services have replaced the country doctor, making house calls and filling the void as rural hospitals have closed.

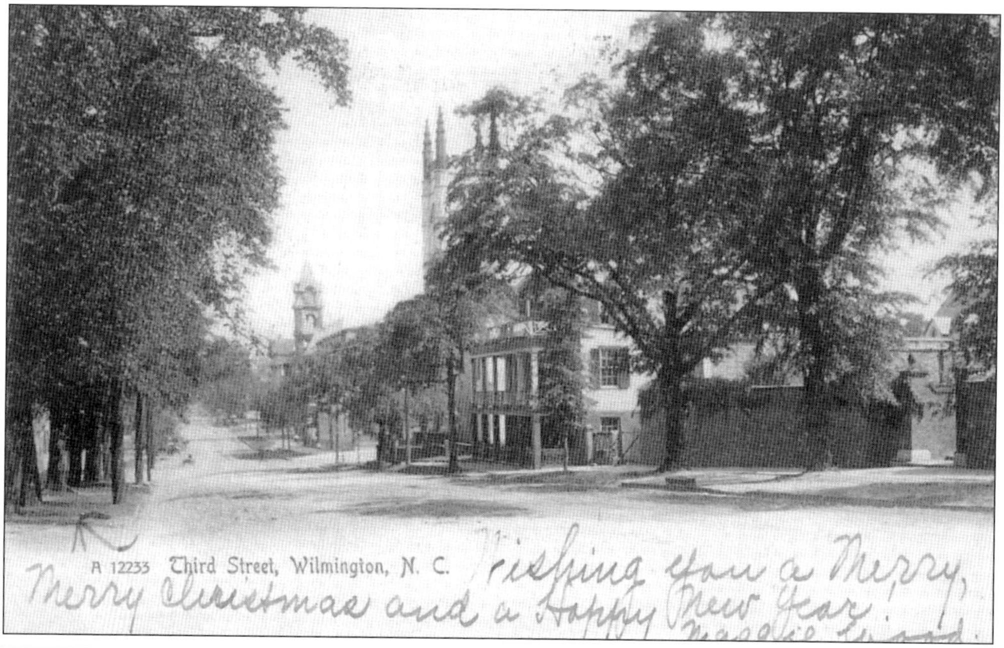

This image from the early 1900s offers a glimpse of Wilmington's past in wartime hospitals and medical education. Looking north on Third Street, the St. James Church is the first tower rising above the trees (at the intersection of Market Street). There, the Union army established a hospital during their 1865 occupation. This building replaced a previous structure on the same site where in 1781, during the occupation by Lord Cornwallis and the British Army, a hospital had been established for their wounded. On the next block, in the distance on the right, is the town hall (100 block of North Third Street). Across the street was the College of Physicians and Surgeons. (New Hanover County Public Library.)

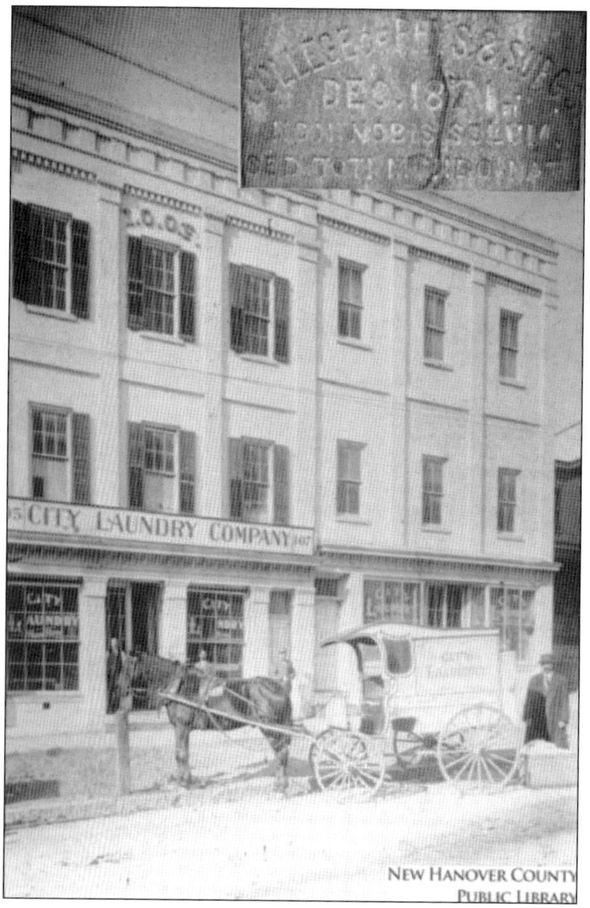

The image to the left is a view of the College of Physicians and Surgeons, which opened in 1871 (albeit briefly closing in 1874). (New Hanover County Public Library.)

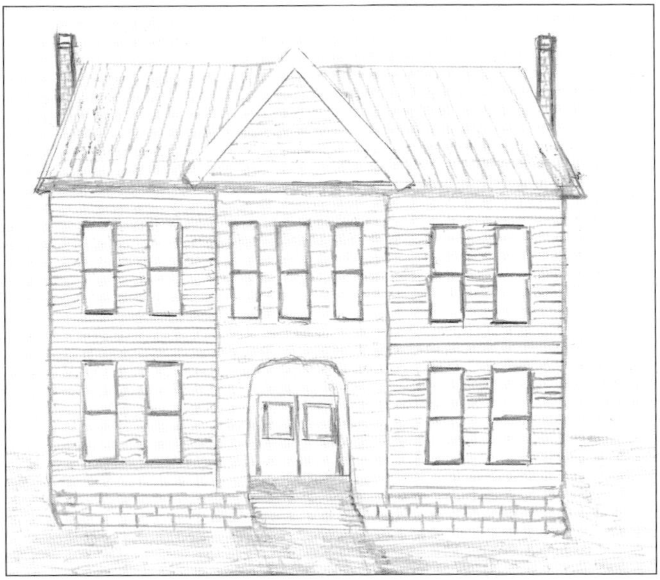

In 1867, North Carolina's first chartered medical school was Edenborough Medical School, located near present-day Raeford (at the time, Robeson County). Dr. Hector McLean was the sole instructor. Dr. McLean, a Scottish descendant, grew up and returned to the area after attending medical school in Louisville. He mentored students before the school was chartered. The school closed upon his death in 1877. (This sketch is based on written descriptions.)

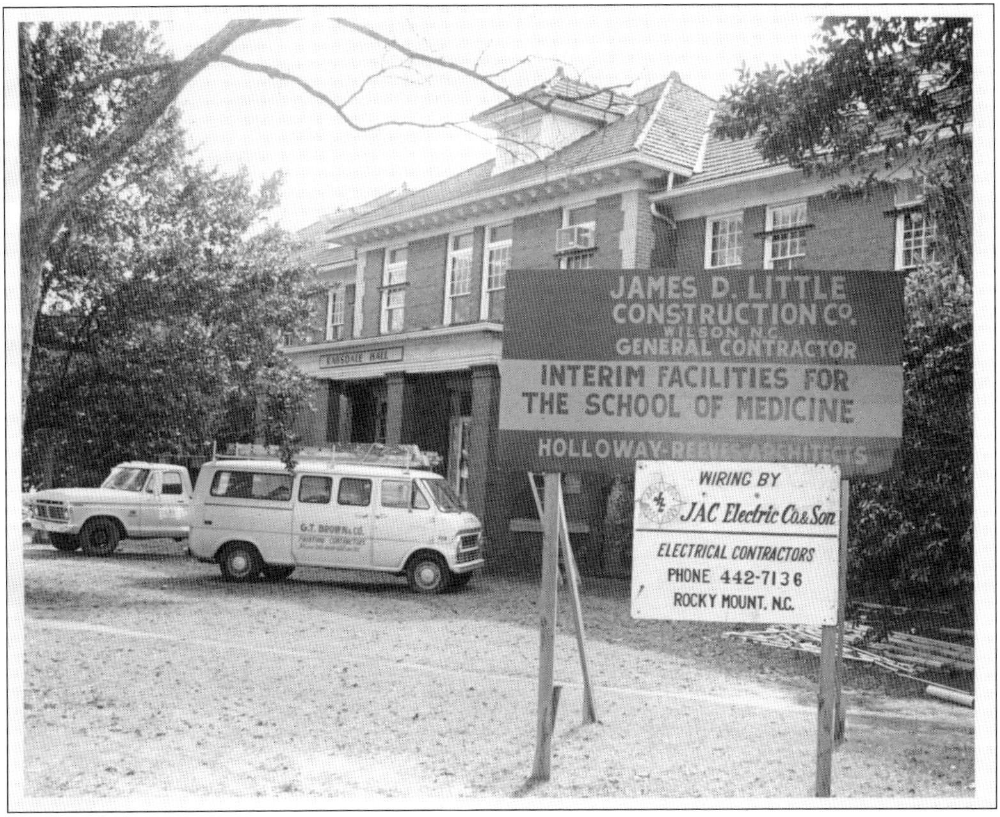
JAMES D. LITTLE
CONSTRUCTION Co.
WILSON N.C.
GENERAL CONTRACTOR
INTERIM FACILITIES FOR
THE SCHOOL OF MEDICINE
WIRING BY
JAC Electric Co.& Son
ELECTRICAL CONTRACTORS
PHONE 442-7136
ROCKY MOUNT, N.C.

The Brody School of Medicine (BSOM) opened in 1977 in Greenville at East Carolina University (ECU). ECU became the second state-sponsored medical school at the time. Today, the school targets students from the rural and coastal region of the state and is ranked as one of the nation's top primary care medical schools. (East Carolina University Digital Collections, Image 22668.)

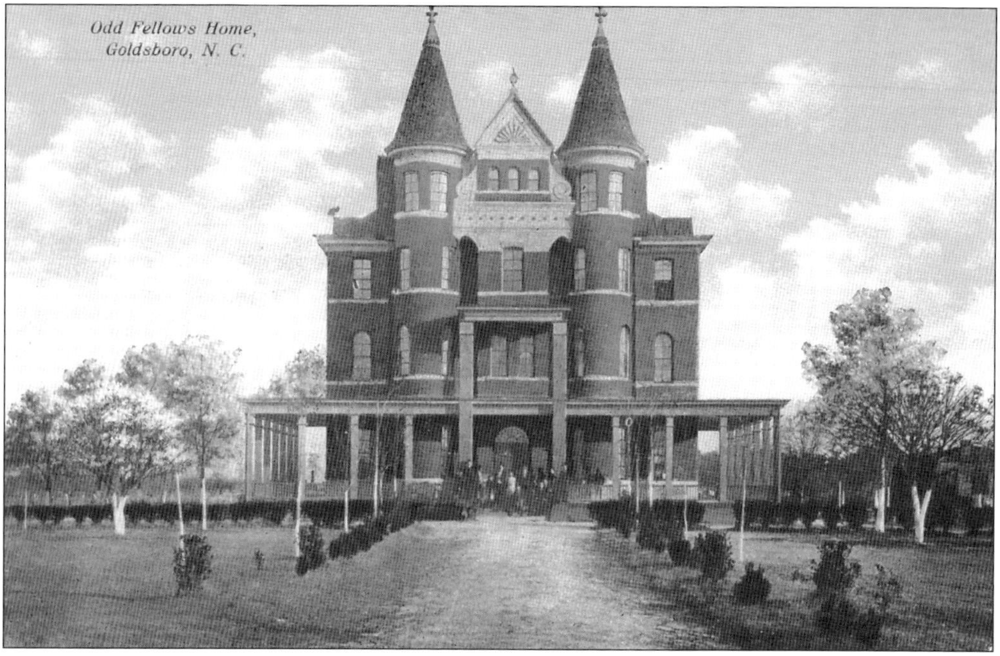

The Odd Fellows Home in Goldsboro opened in 1892 as an orphanage. This massive complex would grow to include residential housing for the elderly (identified as the Old Folks Home) and an infirmary. In 1914, the 126-bed campus identified Leff Wagner as the superintendent. This postcard is an image of the first building.

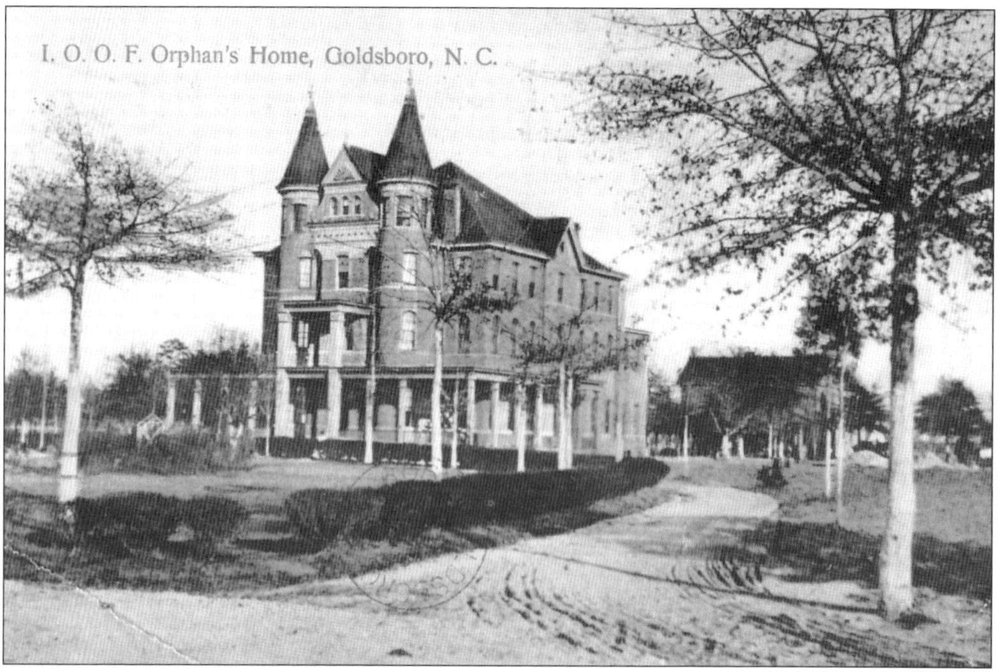

Another view shows the original Odd Fellows building in 1910, located at the corner of North Herman and West Ash Street. It sat across the street from Wayne Memorial Hospital. The Odd Fellows Old Folks Home can be seen in the background.

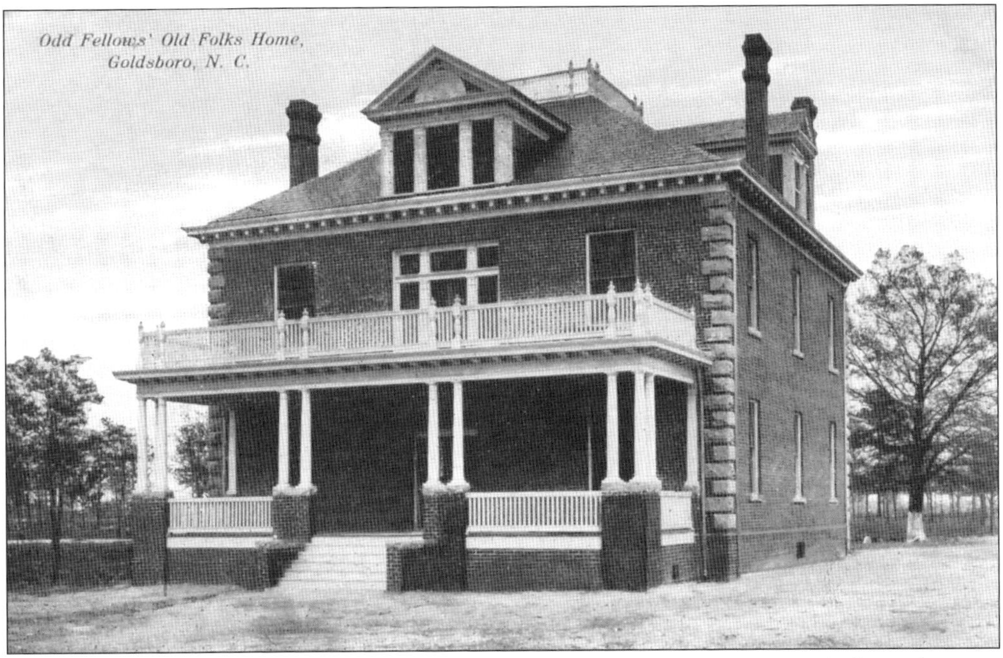

Pictured is a close-up view of the Odd Fellows Old Folks Home on campus with the orphanage. The facility accepted older adults who typically had no means of support.

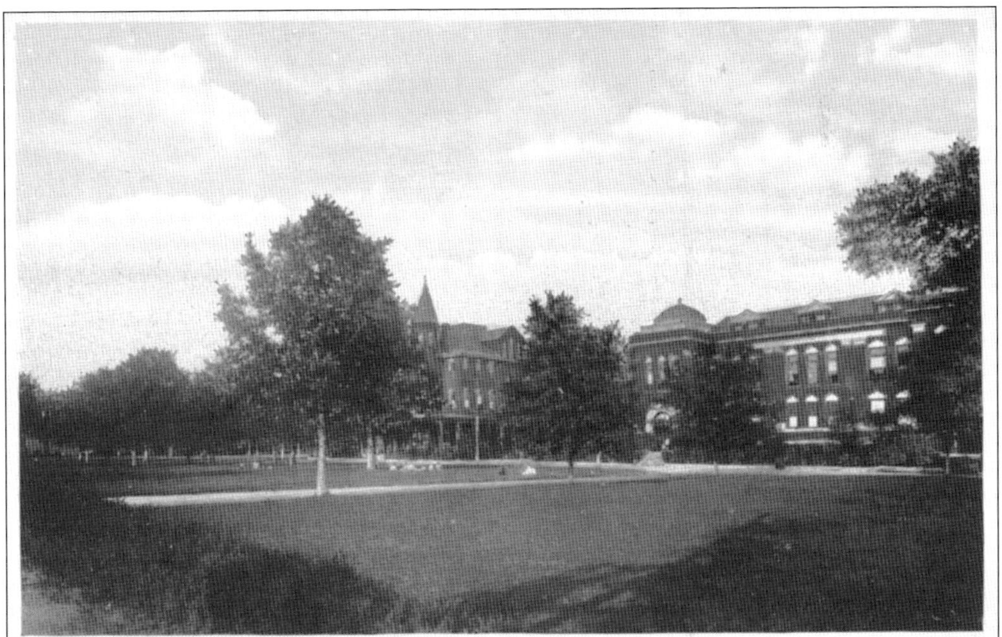

Another view of the Odd Fellows campus in the 1950s offers a glimpse into how truly massive the facility once was. It closed in 1970, and most of the buildings were torn down. Today, the public library occupies part of the former campus property.

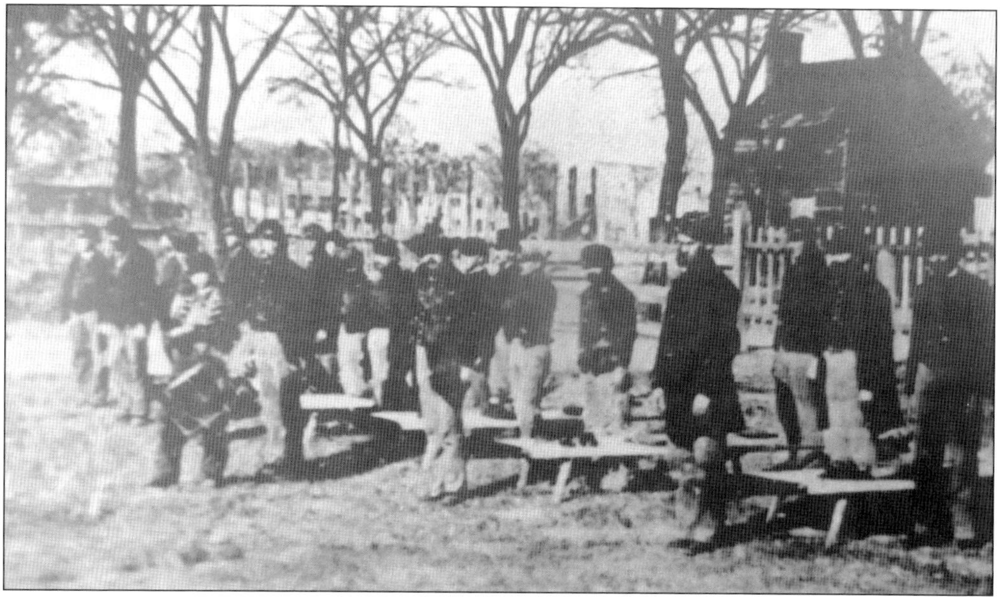

The Stretcher Corps (Union Ambulance Services) is drilling at Newbern around 1863. The men trained to respond rapidly, move a patient to a stretcher, provide whatever care needed, and evacuate the patient to a hospital. The first of the public ambulances emerged following the American Civil War and was based on a model that developed during that war. (US Army Military History Institute.)

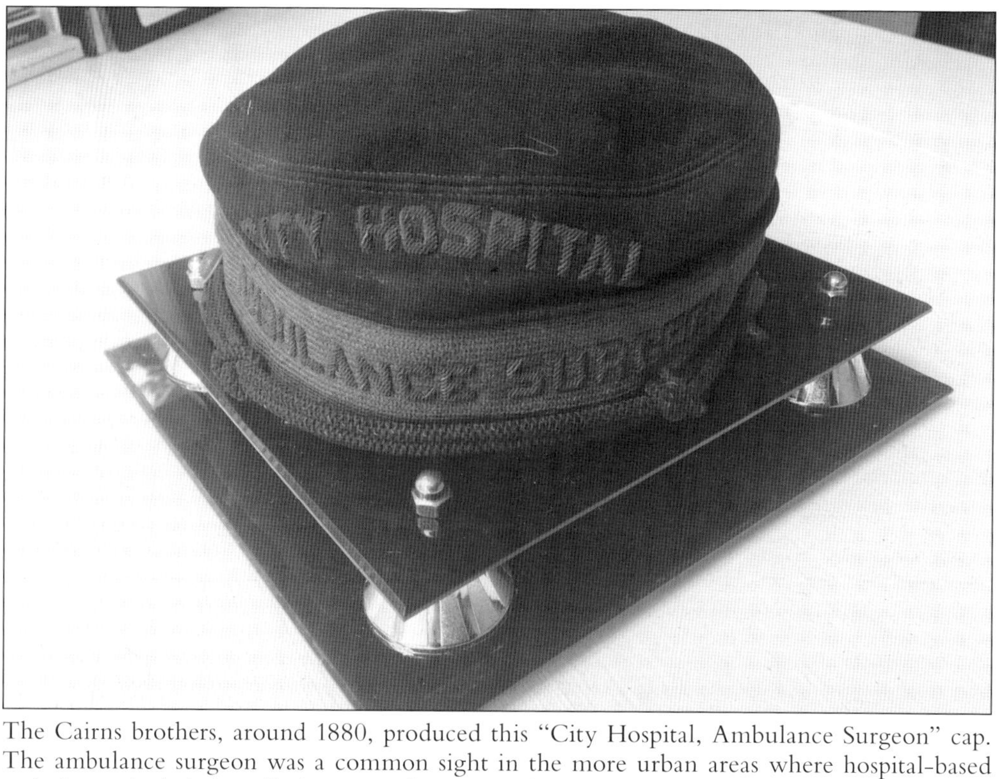

The Cairns brothers, around 1880, produced this "City Hospital, Ambulance Surgeon" cap. The ambulance surgeon was a common sight in the more urban areas where hospital-based ambulances included medical personnel, many with substantial wartime experiences.

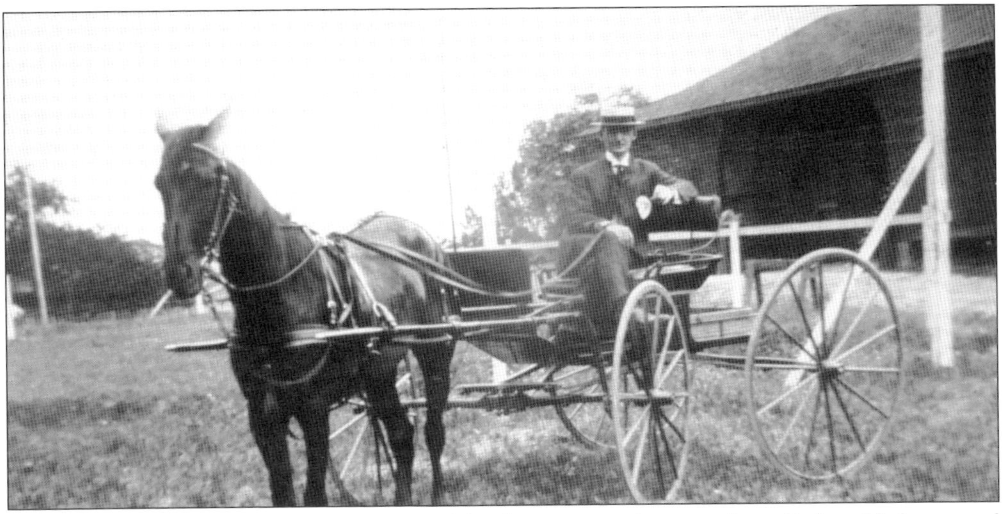

The more rural areas were typically served by the country doctor, who relied on his horse and wagon to make the rounds through the community for the sick and injured. Pictured here is Dr. C.W. Love at the City-County Hospital in Wilmington. Hospitals were typically for those away from home or who lived alone. (New Hanover County Public Library.)

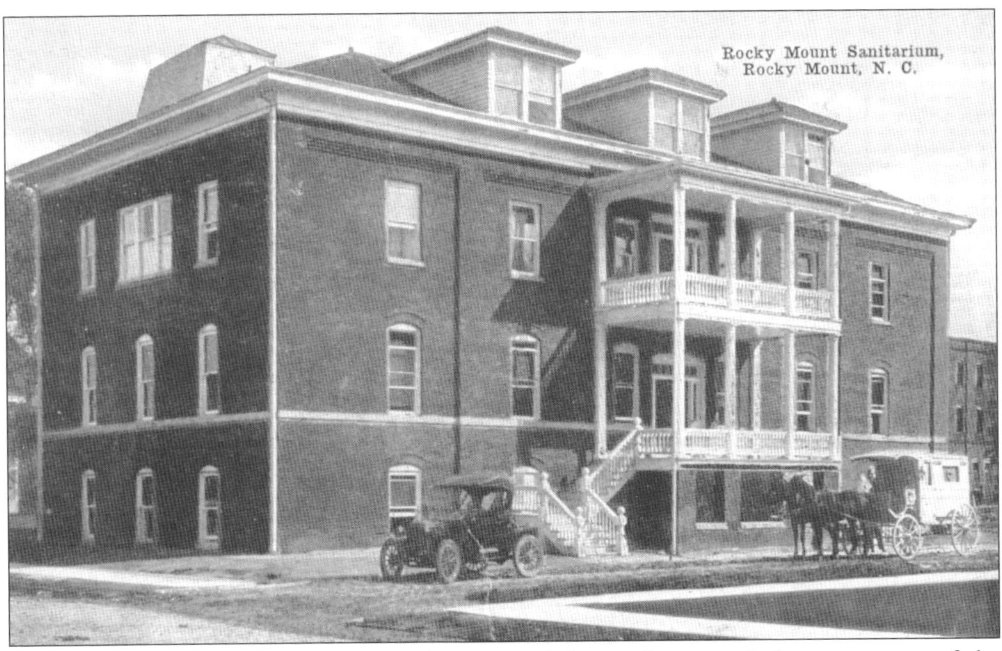

The Rocky Mount Sanitarium opened in 1913. A horse-drawn ambulance was one of the services originally provided by the sanitarium. As residents of a community began to purchase personal automobiles, most hospital-provided ambulances were eliminated.

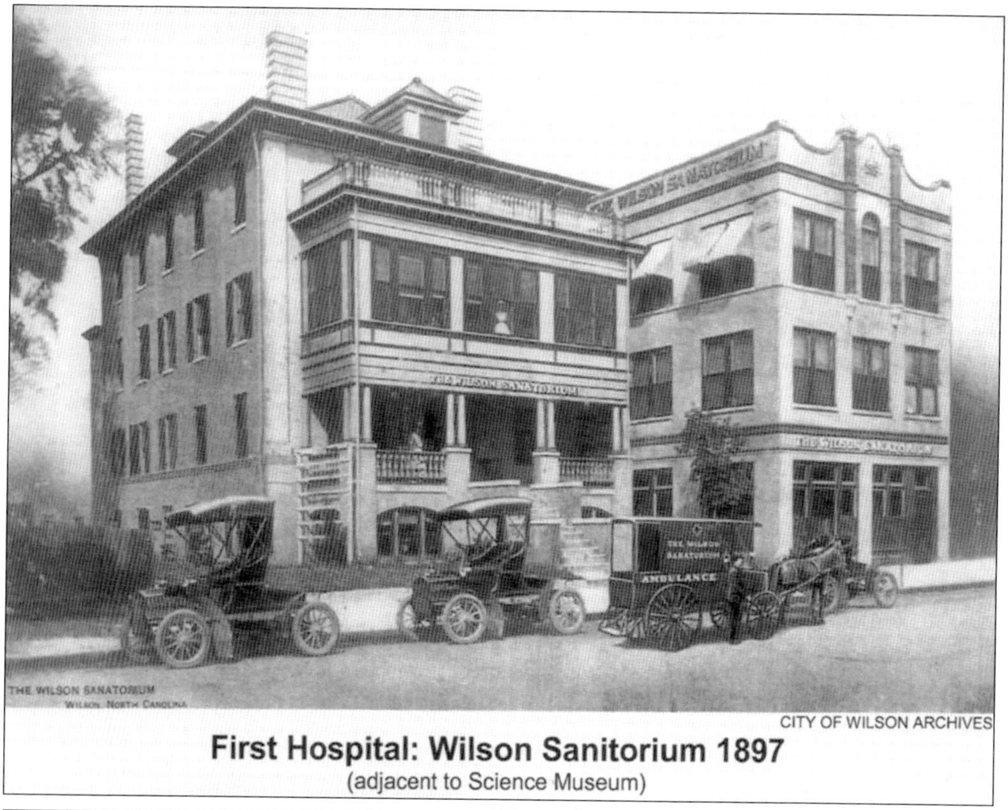
THE WILSON SANATORIUM
WILSON NORTH CAROLINA
AMBULANCE
CITY OF WILSON ARCHIVES
First Hospital: Wilson Sanitorium 1897
(adjacent to Science Museum)

The Wilson Sanitorium opened in 1895. This promotional image of the sanitorium includes its horse-drawn ambulance. (Digital NC, Wilson County Public Library.)

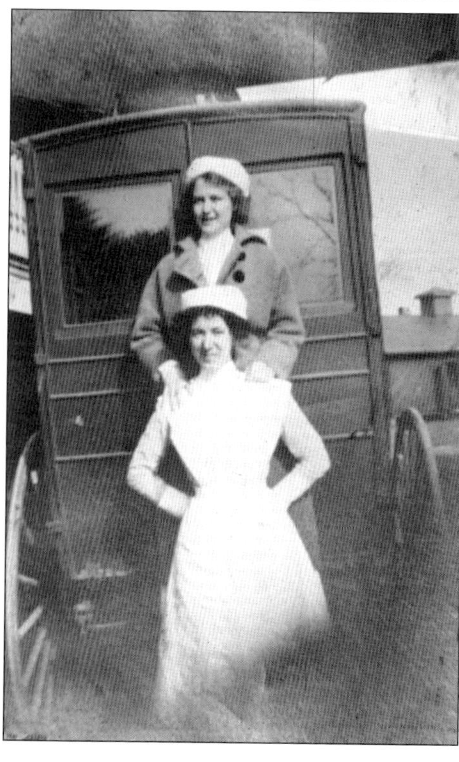

A c. 1905 photograph shows two nurses on the step board of the horse-drawn ambulance at James Walker Memorial Hospital in Wilmington. (New Hanover County Public Library.)

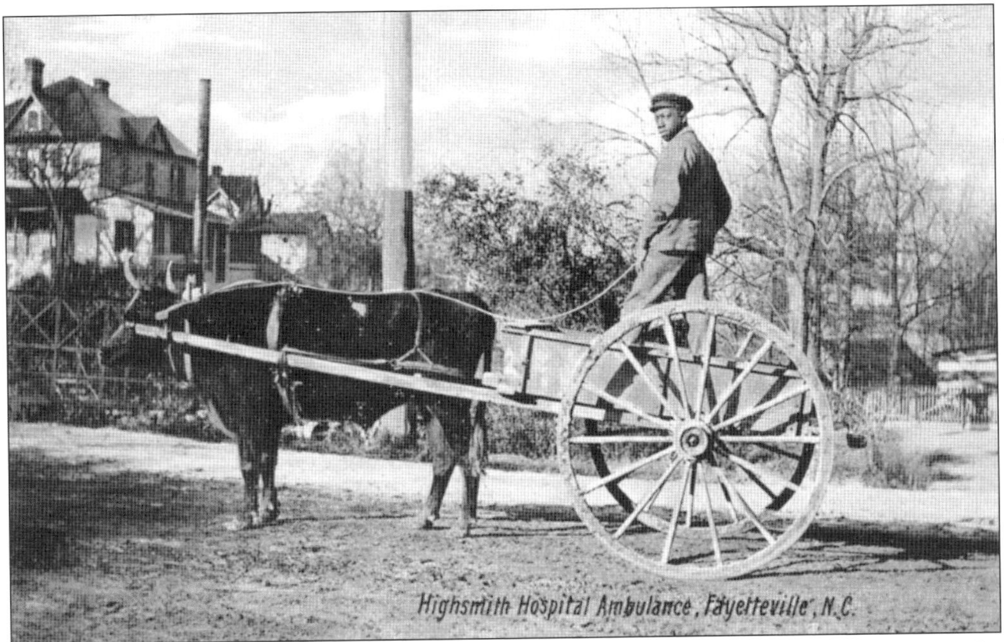

Highsmith Hospital, in Fayetteville, was one of the best equipped and most modern in the South in the early part of the 20th century. This included the Highsmith Hospital ambulance. While it may seem rather crude, the mere fact that the hospital had an ambulance placed it well ahead of most in the context of transportation to the facility.

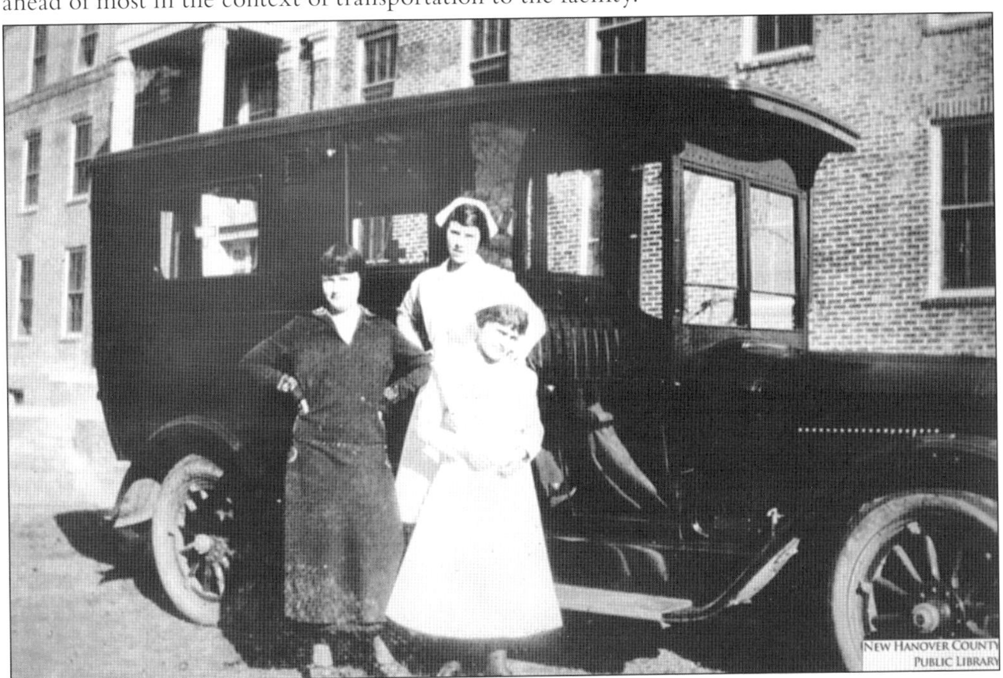

The James Walker Memorial Hospital was one of the first in the state to offer a motorized ambulance service for the community. This ambulance, with nurses, represents an early glimpse into the origins of ambulance and emergency medical services in the state. (New Hanover County Public Library.)

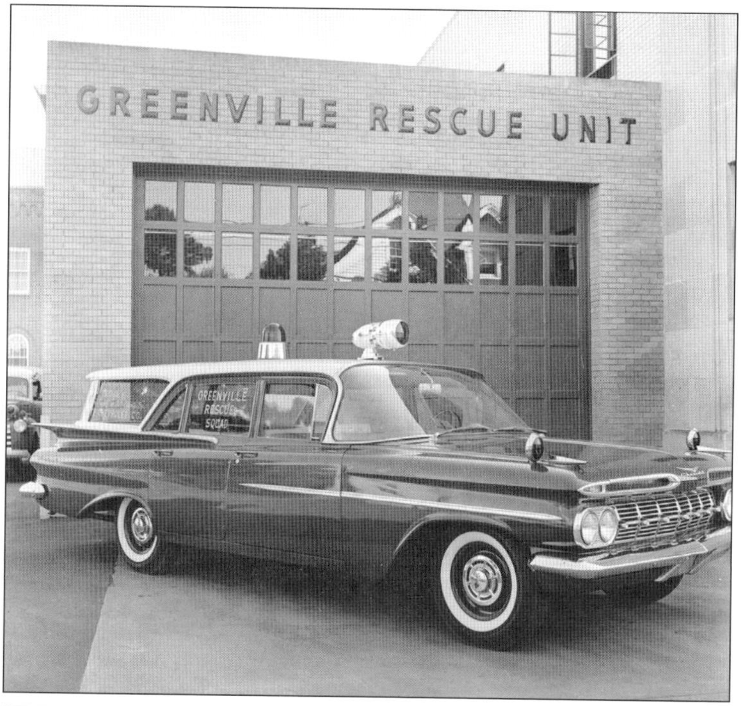

Greenville City Fire and Rescue included this 1960 Chevrolet station wagon ambulance. Greenville Fire and Rescue continues to provide paramedic level EMS today for the city of Greenville. (East Carolina University Digital Collections.)

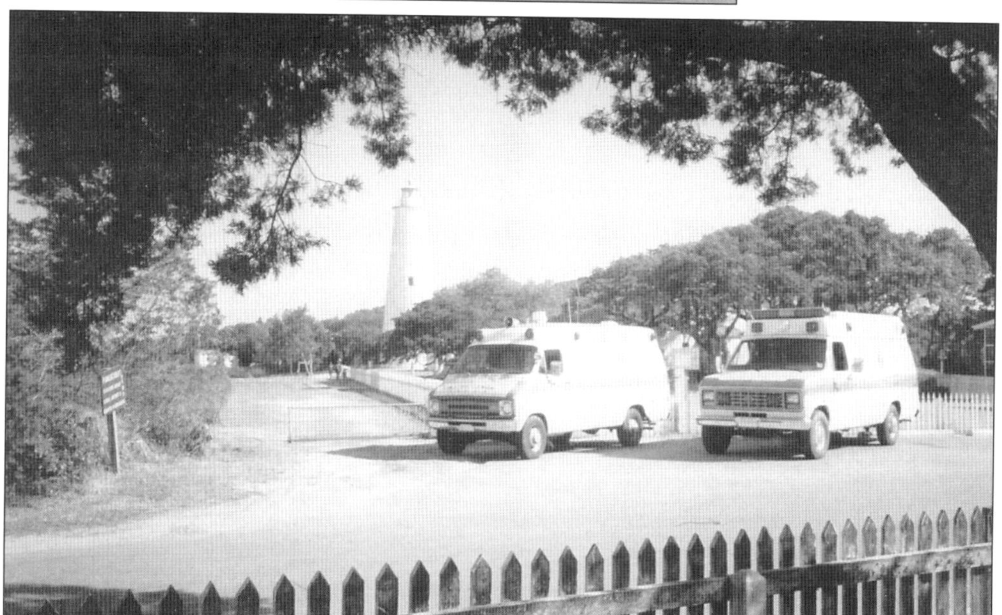

In the early 1800s, Ocracoke Village was the southern tip of Hatteras peninsula, sitting across from Portsmouth Village. Once North Carolina's busiest port, today Ocracoke is one of several barrier islands created when the peninsula was carved up by the 1846 hurricane. Access to Ocracoke is limited to ferry/boat and by air. While there is a clinic, EMS is the only 24-hour medical care. Ambulances pictured here from the 1970s must await the ferry's arrival and travel to the closest hospital several hours away. A weather-dependent alternative is by medical helicopter or airplane.

Postcards were also a common form of communication between the country doctor and places such as the State Agriculture Department. The request pictured here is regarding the testing of a sample that includes suspected typhoid from a physician in Faison.

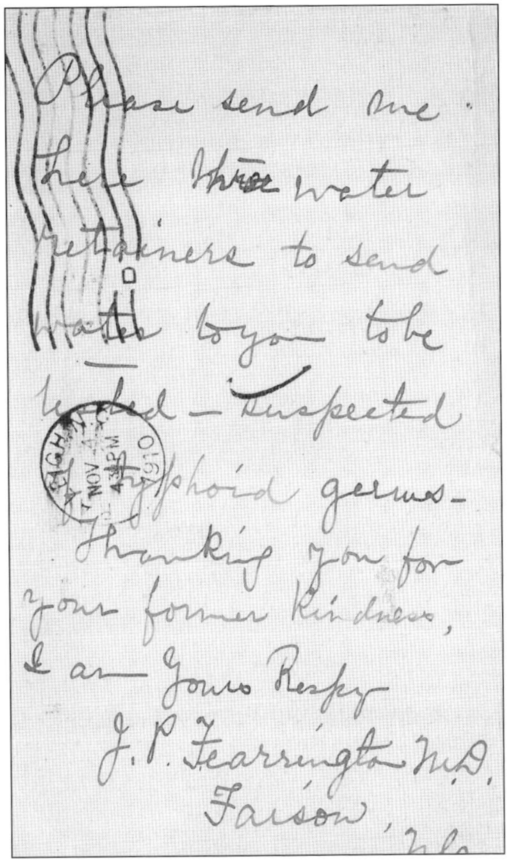

Please send me
here three water
containers to send
water to you to be
tested—suspected
typhoid germs—
Thanking you for
your former kindness,
I am Yours Respy
J. P. Fearrington M.D.
Faison, N.C.

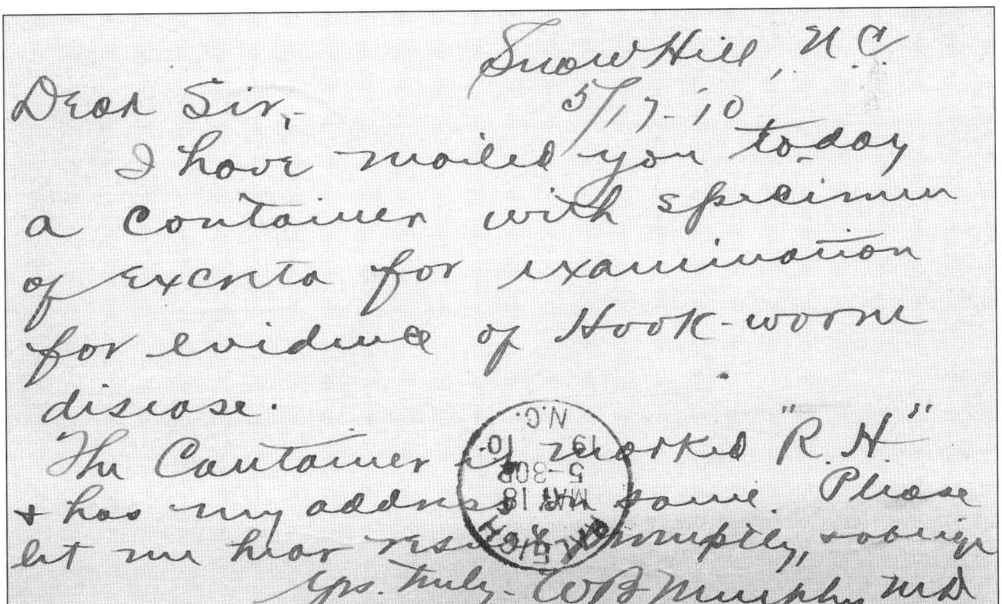

Snow Hill, N.C.
5/17-10
Dear Sir,-
I have mailed you to-day
a container with specimen
of excreta for examination
for evidence of Hook-worm
disease.
The Container is marked "R.H."
+ has my address same. Please
let me hear result promptly, & oblige
Yrs. truly - W. B. Murphy M.D.

Hookworm is suspected in this message from a physician in Snow Hill to the North Carolina Laboratory of Hygiene. These cards created a relatively quick method of sending a message.

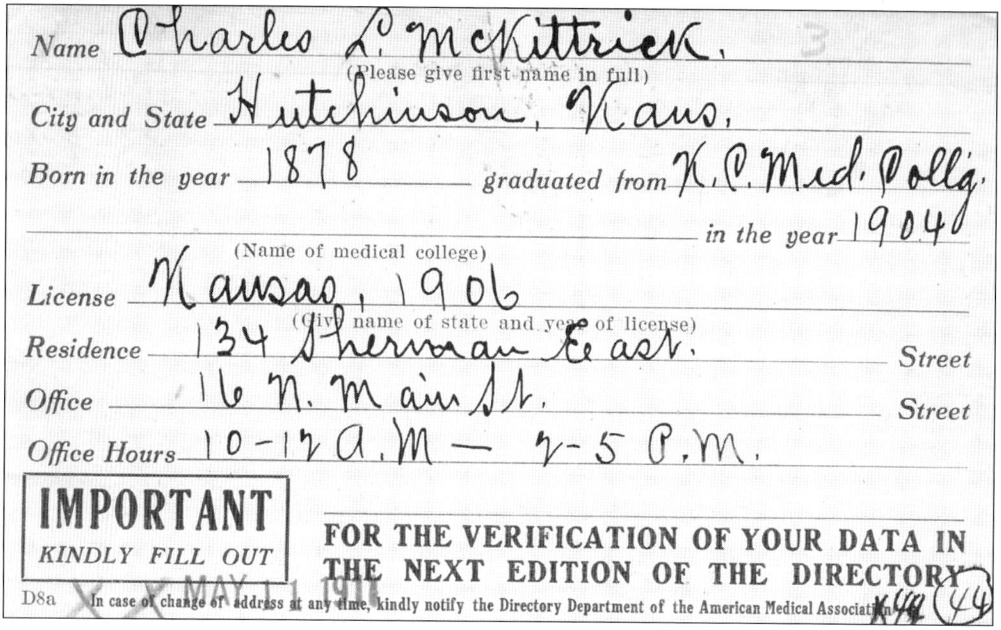

Name Charles L. McKittrick.
(Please give first name in full)

City and State Hutchinson, Kans.

Born in the year 1878 graduated from K. C. Med. Coll'g.

in the year 1904

(Name of medical college)

License Kansas, 1906
(Give name of state and year of license)

Residence 134 Sherman East. Street

Office 16 N. Main St. Street

Office Hours 10-12 A.M — 2-5 P.M.

IMPORTANT
KINDLY FILL OUT

FOR THE VERIFICATION OF YOUR DATA IN THE NEXT EDITION OF THE DIRECTORY

D8a In case of change of address at any time, kindly notify the Directory Department of the American Medical Association.

This postcard from 1911 is an example of a survey sent by the American Medical Association. A Kansas physician participated by filling out the card. A massive, 2,500-plus-page book was created biannually with this information. Those books offered significant details such as locations, specific dates, capacity, and capabilities for specific facilities. This included the superintendent of the facility or, more commonly, the physician in charge (PIC).

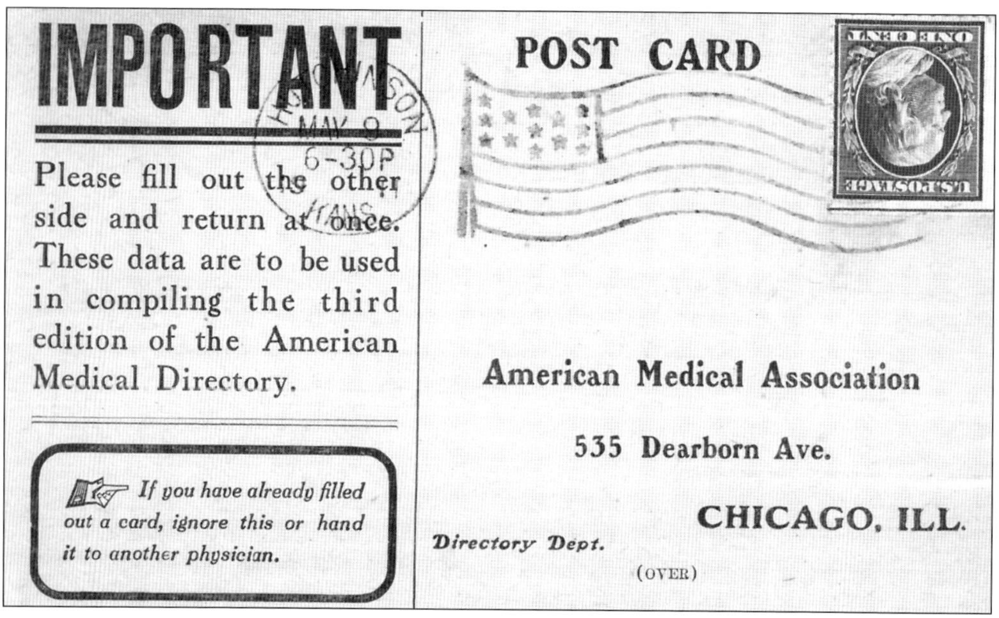

IMPORTANT

Please fill out the other side and return at once. These data are to be used in compiling the third edition of the American Medical Directory.

If you have already filled out a card, ignore this or hand it to another physician.

POST CARD

American Medical Association

535 Dearborn Ave.

CHICAGO, ILL.

Directory Dept.

(OVER)

Bibliography

Adams, H.G. "A Local Chronicle of the Influenza Epidemic of 1918. As Gleaned from Newspaper Accounts of the Day." *North Carolina Medical Journal* 25 (1964): 397–400.

American Medical Association, *American Medical Directory*. A register of physicians of the United States, Alaska, Canal Zone, Hawaii, Philippines, Puerto Rico, Guam, Johnston Island, Virgin Islands and Wake Island, Canada, Newfoundland, Labrador, Yukon, and Northwest Territories. Chicago, IL: Press of American Medical Association, 1906, 1923, 1956.

Daniel, T.M. "The history of tuberculosis." *Respiratory Medicine* 100 (2006):1862–1870.

Eaton, H.A. "Community Hospital, Wilmington, North Carolina: A Historical Account." *Journal of the National Medical Association* 57 (1965): 74–79.

Hardy, Ira L. "What it Costs?" *New Charlotte Medical Journal* 63 (1911): 372–375.

Luchins, A.S. "The Rise and Decline of the American Asylum Movement in the 19th Century."*The Journal of Psychology* 122 (1988): 471–486.

Noah, V.B. "The effect of the Flexner report on North Carolina medical schools." *North Carolina Medical Journal* 26 (1965): 537–541.

Perrone, L.A., and T.M. Tumpey. "Reconstruction of the 1918 pandemic influenza virus: how revealing the molecular secrets of the virus responsible for the worst pandemic in recorded history can guide our response to future influenza pandemics." *Infect Disord Drug Targets* 7 (2007): 294–303.

"Principal Hospitals in the Confederate States." *Confederate States Medical and Surgical Journal* 1 (1864): 129–152.

Rozear, M.P. 1991. "Historical note: North Carolina's first hospital." *North Carolina Medical Journal* 52 (1991): 271–274.

Report of the State Hospital at Goldsboro, NC from November 30, 1902, to November 30, 1904. Raleigh, NC: E.M. Uzzell & Co., State Printers and Binders, 1905.

"The Community Hospital, Wilmington, NC." *Journal of the National Medical Association* 15 (1923): 114.

"The Hill-Burton Bill." *American Journal of Public Health and the Nation's Health* 35 (1945): 380.

US Department of Health, Education, and Welfare. *Storage Locations: Pre-positioned and Training Civil Defense Emergency Hospitals.* Washington, DC: US Government Printing Office, 1964.